Youth Sports Concussions

Guest Editors

KATHLEEN R. BELL, MD
STANLEY A. HERRING, MD

PHYSICAL MEDICINE AND REHABILITATION CLINICS OF NORTH AMERICA

www.pmr.theclinics.com

Consulting Editor
GEORGE H. KRAFT, MD, MS

November 2011 • Volume 22 • Number 4

SAUNDERS an imprint of ELSEVIER, Inc.

W.B. SAUNDERS COMPANY
A Division of Elsevier Inc.

1600 John F. Kennedy Boulevard • Suite 1800 • Philadelphia, Pennsylvania 19103

http://www.theclinics.com

PHYSICAL MEDICINE AND REHABILITATION CLINICS OF NORTH AMERICA Volume 22, Number 4
November 2011 ISSN 1047-9651, ISBN-13: 978-1-4557-7989-5

Editor: David Parsons

Reprints. For copies of 100 or more of articles in this publication, please contact the Commercial Reprints Department, Elsevier Inc., 360 Park Avenue South, New York, NY 10010-1710. Tel.: 212-633-3812; Fax: 212-462-1935; E-mail: reprints@elsevier.com.

Physical Medicine and Rehabilitation Clinics of North America (ISSN 1047-9651) is published quarterly by Elsevier Inc., 360 Park Avenue South, New York, NY 10010-1710. Months of issue are February, May, August, and November. Business and Editorial Offices: 1600 John F. Kennedy Blvd., Suite 1800, Philadelphia, PA 19103-2899. Customer Service Office: 3251 Riverport Lane, Maryland Heights, MO 63043. Periodicals postage paid at New York, NY and additional mailing offices. Subscription price per year is $230.00 (US individuals), $414.00 (US institutions), $122.00 (US students), $280.00 (Canadian individuals), $540.00 (Canadian institutions), $175.00 (Canadian students), $345.00 (foreign individuals), $540.00 (foreign institutions), and $175.00 (foreign students). Foreign air speed delivery is included in all *Clinics* subscription prices. All prices are subject to change without notice. **POSTMASTER:** Send address changes to *Physical Medicine and Rehabilitation Clinics of North America*, Customer Service Office: Elsevier Health Sciences Division, Subscription Customer Service, 3251 Riverport Lane, Maryland Heights, MO 63043. **Customer Service: 1-800-654-2452 (US). From outside of the United States, call 314-447-8871. Fax: 314-447-8029. E-mail: JournalsCustomer Service-usa@elsevier.com (for print support); JournalsOnlineSupport-usa@elsevier.com (for online support).**

Physical Medicine and Rehabilitation Clinics of North America is indexed in *Excerpta Medica, MEDLINE/ PubMed (Index Medicus), Cinahl,* and *Cumulative Index to Nursing and Allied Health Literature.*

Printed and bound by CPI Group (UK) Ltd, Croydon, CR0 4YY

Transferred to Digital Print 2011

Contributors

CONSULTING EDITOR

GEORGE H. KRAFT, MD
Alvord Professor of Multiple Sclerosis Research; Professor, Department of Rehabilitation Medicine, and Adjunct Professor, Department of Neurology, University of Washington, Seattle, Washington

GUEST EDITORS

KATHLEEN R. BELL, MD
Professor, Department of Rehabilitation Medicine; Director, Traumatic Brain Injury Model System, University of Washington, Seattle, Washington

STANLEY A. HERRING, MD
Clinical Professor, Departments of Rehabilitation Medicine, Orthopaedics and Sports Medicine and Neurological Surgery, University of Washington; Co-Medical Director Seattle Sports Concussion Program, Team Physician Seattle Seahawks and Seattle Mariners, Seattle, Washington

AUTHORS

RICHARD H. ADLER, JD
Attorney at Law, Founding Principal of Adler Giersch, P.S. Law Firm, Chairman, Executive Board, Brain Injury Association of Washington, Seattle, Washington

KATHLEEN R. BELL, MD
Professor, Department of Rehabilitation Medicine; Director, Traumatic Brain Injury Model System, University of Washington, Seattle, Washington

HEIDI K. BLUME, MD, MPH
Assistant Professor of Neurology, Division of Pediatric Neurology, Seattle Children's Hospital, University of Washington, Seattle, Washington

STEVEN P. BROGLIO, PhD, ATC
School of Kinesiology, University of Michigan, Ann Arbor, Michigan

ROBERT C. CANTU, MD
Co-Director, Department of Neurology, Center for the Study of Traumatic Encephalopathy (CSTE), Boston University School of Medicine (BUSM); Co-Founder, Sports Legacy Institute, Waltham, Massachusetts; Co-Director, Neurologic Sports Injury Center, Brigham and Women's Hospital, Boston, Massachusetts; Director of Sports Medicine, Chief of Neurosurgery Service, Chairman, Department of Surgery, Emerson Hospital; Clinical Professor, Department of Neurosurgery, Center for the Study of Traumatic Encephalopathy (CSTE), Boston University School of Medicine (BUSM), Concord, Massachusetts

DAVID B. COPPEL, PhD
Professor, Department of Neurological Surgery, University of Washington; Director of Neuropsychological Services and Research, Seattle Sports Concussion Program, Harborview Medical Center and Seattle Children's Medical Center, Seattle, Washington

DANIEL H. DANESHVAR, MA
Graduate Student, Department of Neurology, Center for the Study of Traumatic Encephalopathy (CSTE), Boston University School of Medicine (BUSM), Boston, Massachusetts

GERARD A. GIOIA, PhD
Chief, Division of Pediatric Neuropsychology; Director, Safe Concussion Outcome, Recovery & Education (SCORE) Program, Children's National Medical Center, Rockville, Maryland; Associate Professor, Departments of Psychiatry & Behavioral Sciences and Pediatrics, The George Washington University School of Medicine, Washington, DC

CHRISTOPHER C. GIZA, MD
Division of Pediatric Neurology, Department of Pediatrics, David Geffen School of Medicine at UCLA, Mattel Children's Hospital, UCLA, Los Angeles; Department of Neurosurgery, UCLA Brain Injury Research Center, Semel Institute, David Geffen School of Medicine at UCLA, Los Angeles, California

GRACE S. GRIESBACH, PhD
Adjunct Assistant Professor, Department of Neurosurgery, UCLA Brain Injury Research Center, Semel Institute, David Geffen School of Medicine at UCLA, Los Angeles, California

KEVIN M. GUSKIEWICZ, PhD, ATC
Department of Exercise and Sport Science, University of North Carolina at Chapel Hill, Chapel Hill, North Carolina

JEFFREY G. JARVIK, MD, MPH
Faculty, Departments of Radiology, Neurological Surgery, and Health Services; Director, Comparative Effectiveness, Cost and Outcomes Research Center, University of Washington, Seattle, Washington

THOMAS M. JINGUJI, MD
Attending Physician, Clinical Assistant Professor, Department of Orthopedics and Sports Medicine, Seattle Children's Hospital, University of Washington, Seattle, Washington

BRIAN J. KRABAK, MD, MBA
Clinical Associate Professor, University of Washington and Seattle Children's Sports Medicine; Physician, University of Washington and Seattle University Athletics; Medical Director, Racing The Planet Ultramarathons, Seattle, Washington

SCOTT R. LAKER, MD
Assistant Professor, Department of Physical Medicine and Rehabilitation, University of Colorado, Aurora, Colorado

SYLVIA LUCAS, MD, PhD
Clinical Professor of Neurology, Adjunct Clinical Professor of Rehabilitation Medicine, University of Washington; Director, University of Washington Headache Center, Seattle Washington

BRENDAN J. MCCULLOUGH, MD, PhD
Department of Radiology, Comparative Effectiveness, Cost and Outcomes Research Center, University of Washington, Seattle, Washington

ANN C. MCKEE, MD
Co-Director, Associate Professor of Neurology and Pathology, Department of Neurology, Center for the Study of Traumatic Encephalopathy (CSTE), Bedford VA Hospital, Boston University School of Medicine (BUSM), Boston, Massachusetts

CHRISTOPHER J. NOWINSKI, AB
Co-Director, Department of Neurology, Center for the Study of Traumatic Encephalopathy (CSTE), Boston University School of Medicine (BUSM), Boston; Co-Founder, Sports Legacy Institute, Waltham, Massachusetts

DAVID O. RILEY, SB
Research Assistant, Department of Neurology, Center for the Study of Traumatic Encephalopathy (CSTE), Boston University School of Medicine (BUSM), Boston, Massachusetts

MAEGAN D. SADY, PhD
Postdoctoral Fellow, Division of Pediatric Neuropsychology, Children's National Medical Center, Rockville, Maryland

EMMA K. SATCHELL
Research Associate, Seattle Children's Hospital, Seattle, Washington

DANIEL W. SHREY, MD
Fellow Physician, Division of Pediatric Neurology, Department of Pediatrics, David Geffen School of Medicine at UCLA, Mattel Children's Hospital, UCLA, Los Angeles, California

ROBERT A. STERN, PhD
Co-Director, Associate Professor of Neurology, Department of Neurology, Center for the Study of Traumatic Encephalopathy (CSTE), Boston University School of Medicine (BUSM), Boston, Massachusetts

CHRISTOPHER G. VAUGHAN, PsyD
Pediatric Neuropsychologist, Division of Pediatric Neuropsychology, Children's National Medical Center, Rockville, Maryland; Assistant Professor, Departments of Psychiatry & Behavioral Sciences and Pediatrics, The George Washington University School of Medicine, Washington, DC

Contents

Concussions occur as a result of forces directed to the head or neck, or from impulsive forces transmitted from the body to the head. They result in the rapid onset and spontaneous recovery of short-lived impairment of neurologic function. Concussions represent a functional, rather than structural, disturbance, and do not result in abnormalities on standard structural imaging. This article discusses a comprehensive approach to return to play in sports concussion, including managing athletes returning after prolonged postconcussion syndrome, multiple concussions, and intracranial hematomas and craniotomy.

The primary role of neuroimaging in the clinical context of sports-related concussion is the exclusion of a more severe, unsuspected intracranial injury. Computed tomography remains the test of choice for this purpose. Magnetic resonance imaging is more commonly used as a secondary test for the investigation of persistent symptoms. New imaging techniques are currently being developed to detect the molecular and cellular changes underlying concussion that are invisible with standard structural imaging. In the future, these techniques may be used as tools for directing rehabilitation after concussion and aiding in the decision of when it is safe for an athlete to return to play.

Neuropsychological or neurocognitive tests provide information regarding the cognitive and emotional status of the concussed athlete. The development and availability of computerized testing platforms has allowed the application of baseline and follow-up testing models, and provide a more precise measurement of reaction time and processing speed. A combination of computerized assessment and a more expanded battery of tests may be a better approach to understanding the nature of the cognitive impact of sports concussion in youth athletes. This approach may be especially important for athletes with general risk factors and other potential modifiers or influencers on the cognitive performance data.

Most athletes who experience a sports-related concussion recover from the acute effects within a few weeks. However, some children and adolescents with concussion experience symptoms for many weeks, or even months after the injury. Subacute and chronic symptoms related to concussion are particularly concerning in children, because cognitive deficits, headache or neck pain, sleep dysfunction, and emotional dysregulation can affect school performance and social function at a critical period of development and maturation. This article reviews the epidemiology of subacute symptoms after pediatric concussion and the current recommendations for the assessment and management of these symptoms in children and adolescents.

Each year in the United States, approximately 1.7 million people are diagnosed with a traumatic brain injury (TBI), about 75% of which are classified as mild TBIs or concussions. Although symptoms typically resolve in a matter of weeks, both children and adults may suffer from postconcussion syndrome for months or longer. A progressive tauopathy, chronic traumatic encephalopathy, is believed to stem from repeated brain trauma. Alzheimer-like dementia, Parkinsonism, and motor neuron disease are also associated with repetitive brain trauma. Effective diagnoses, treatments, and education plans are required to reduce the future burden and incidence of long-term effects of head injuries.

School learning and performance is arguably the critical centerpiece of child and adolescent development, and there can be significant temporary upset in cognitive processing after a mild traumatic brain injury, also called a concussion. This injury results in a cascade of neurochemical abnormalities, and, in the wake of this dysfunction, both physical and cognitive activities become sources of additional neurometabolic demand on the brain and may cause symptoms to reemerge or worsen. This article provides a foundation for postinjury management of cognitive activity, particularly in the school setting, including design and implementation of schoolwide concussion education and management programs.

Effective concussion prevention and management for youth athletes requires both education and legislation. Education alone effectively begins the awareness of an issue, but does not change behavior. Education and legislation are required to prevent preventable concussion and brain injuries in youth athletes.

FORTHCOMING ISSUE

THE CLINICS ARE NOW AVAILABLE ONLINE!

Access your subscription at:
www.theclinics.com

Preface

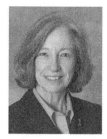 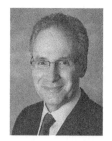

Kathleen R. Bell, MD   Stanley A. Herring, MD
Guest Editors

A teacher affects eternity; he can never tell where his influence stops.
—*Adams, Henry. The Education of Henry Adams, 1918.*

First things first. We are honored to have been asked to guest edit this volume of *Physical Medicine and Rehabilitation of North America*, the final issue directed by George H. Kraft, MD, our friend and teacher. Dr Kraft has been the consulting editor for this esteemed journal since 1990 and, in doing so, has extended his teaching and influence to a national and international audience. We cannot thank him enough for his mentoring and guidance throughout the years.

We were excited at the opportunity to develop this volume addressing Youth Sports Concussion. As physiatrists, we are devoted to caring for people with acute and chronic disorders that affect daily abilities, including work, school, family life, and yes, sports. Often the topic of sports-related concussion is narrowly addressed. With the backdrop of our training in physical medicine and rehabilitation, and our individual practices as a sports physician and a brain injury specialist, we tried to bring together the experts who could discuss the full spectrum of sports-related concussions in youth athletes, from on the field management to school performance to ongoing health problems. It is important for athletes, parents, coaches, athletic trainers, physicians, and others to understand that concussion may not only be a single event. Recovery from concussion, especially repeated insults, is an ongoing process that may require expert management over a more extended period of time than is often considered.

Taking into account these issues, we gathered authorities from many venues. Drs Thomas Jinguji and colleagues review the epidemiology of youth sports concussions, and Dr Christopher Giza and his group explore how the pathophysiology of concussion is different in the developing brain. Acute management of concussion and return to play decisions are discussed by Drs Kevin Guskiewicz, Steven Broglio, and Scott Laker. The third section of this volume covers the current state of diagnosis for

Phys Med Rehabil Clin N Am 22 (2011) xi–xii
doi:10.1016/j.pmr.2011.08.011

concussion with articles on neuroimaging by Drs McCullough and Jarvik and neuro-psychological testing by Dr Coppel. The longer term consequences of concussion in children form the fourth section. Drs Blume, Lucas, and Bell discuss the subacute medical problems in children and Dr Cantu and his colleagues review the long-term neuropathologic consequences of concussion on the young brain. Finally, our last section examines community responses to youth sports concussion. Dr Goia and associates review how concussion might affect school performance and the need for educational management. A blueprint for legislative action, as exemplified by the Washington state Lystedt law regulating early management of youth sports-related concussion, is given by Mr Richard Adler. Thank you to all authors for finding the time in unforgiving schedules to produce such quality work.

We are encouraged and gratified by the attention and enthusiasm of the medical and public community to addressing this preventable and treatable disorder, and we offer our thanks to Zackery Lystedt and his parents, Victor and Mercedes, for their endless courage and determination, a sustaining source of inspiration for us all.

Kathleen R. Bell, MD
Department of Rehabilitation Medicine
University of Washington
Traumatic Brain Injury Model Systems
1959 NE Pacific Street
Seattle, WA 98195, USA

Stanley A. Herring, MD
Departments of Rehabilitation Medicine
Orthopaedics and Sports Medicine and Neurological Surgery
University of Washington
4225 Roosevelt Way, NE
Seattle, WA 98105, USA

E-mail addresses:
krbell@u.washington.edu (K.R. Bell)
sherring@u.washington.edu (S.A. Herring)

Dedication

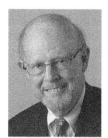

George Kraft

Elsevier would like to thank Dr George Kraft for his more than twenty years serving as the Consulting Editor for *Physical Medicine and Rehabilitation Clinics of North America*. This is Dr Kraft's final issue as Consulting Editor for the Clinics. His time and effort have been paramount to our growth over the years, and we wish him all the best in his future endeavors.

Phys Med Rehabil Clin N Am 22 (2011) xiii
doi:10.1016/j.pmr.2011.09.001
1047-9651/11/$ – see front matter © 2011 Elsevier Inc. All rights reserved.

Epidemiology of Youth Sports Concussion

Thomas M. Jinguji, MD[a,b,*], Brian J. Krabak, MD, MBA[c,d,e], Emma K. Satchell[b]

KEYWORDS

• Concussion • High school athletes • Head injury • Youth

SPORTS CONCUSSION

Estimates of the frequency of sports concussion are truly estimates. Before 2006, an often quoted number for total sports-related concussion in the United States was 300,000 per year. This number is based on data from 1991 National Health Interview Survey in which 46,700 households (120,000 persons) were interviewed, and, from these data, it was estimated that 1.54 million mild head injuries occurred in the year 1990 in the United States. Around 20% of these injuries occurred during sports or physical activity. To be counted as mild, the head injury had to involve loss of consciousness but did not have to be severe enough to cause death or long-term institutionalization.[1] Estimates of sports concussion causing loss of consciousness range between 8% and 19.2%.[2,3] Based on these data, Langlois and colleagues[4] estimated sports concussion at 1.6 million to 3.8 million events per year in the United States. This is an estimate of all sports concussion in the United States and does not address any specific age group.

YOUTH SPORTS CONCUSSION

On May 20, 2010 the US Government Accountability Office (GAO) gave testimony before the House Committee on Education and Labor regarding the occurrence of concussion in high school sports. The GAO believed that the "overall estimate of occurrence is not available."[5] Multiple definitions for concussion, poor recognition

These authors have nothing to disclose.
[a] Department of Orthopedics and Sports Medicine, University of Washington, Seattle, WA, USA
[b] Seattle Children's, W-7706 – Orthopedics Administration, 4800 And Point Way NE, Seattle, WA 98105, USA
[c] University of Washington and Seattle Children's Sports Medicine, Seattle, WA, USA
[d] University of Washington and Seattle University Athletics, Seattle, WA, USA
[e] RacingThePlanet Ultramarathons, Seattle, WA, USA
* Corresponding author. Seattle Children's, W-7706 – Orthopedics Administration, 4800 And Point Way NE, Seattle, WA 98105.
E-mail address: Thomas.Jinguji@seattlechildrens.org

Phys Med Rehabil Clin N Am 22 (2011) 565–575
doi:10.1016/j.pmr.2011.08.001
1047-9651/11/$ – see front matter © 2011 Elsevier Inc. All rights reserved.

of this condition, and underreporting in the high school setting lead to the assumption that concussion is probably underestimated in youth sports.[6]

Yard and Comstock[7] studied 100 high schools for more than 3 years and found 1308 concussions during 5,627,921 athletic exposures (AE). From this study, they estimated 395, 274 concussions per year in US high school athletes from 9 sports. There have been estimates that sport-related concussion accounts for approximately 9% of high school athletic injuries (**Fig. 1**).[8]

GENERAL CONSIDERATIONS

It is well documented that high school athletes with concussions take longer to recover than collegiate and adult athletes.[9,10]

Adults and professional athletes usually recover relatively quickly from concussion with cognitive testing returning to baseline within 3 to 5 days of initial injury. College athletes show an average recovery time of 5 to 7 days. High school athletes take even longer to heal, with average recovery times of 10 to 14 days.[6]

Concussions in high school sports occur much more frequently in games than during practice. The only sport that shows a higher concussion rate in practice than competition is cheerleading.[3] Also, for sports in which both sexes participate, reported concussion rates are higher for female than male high school athletes. Recent data show that the time required for return to play and resolution of symptoms is similar for girls and boys.[11]

Very little is known about the epidemiology of concussions in middle school–aged athletes and younger children. An emergency department (ED) surveillance study from 2001 to 2005 estimated 253,000 ED visits for sports concussion for the age range 8 to 19 years. Around 40% (approximately 102,000 visits) were in the age range 8 to 13 years, and the remaining 60% (151,000) were in the 14- to 19-year range. In those aged 8 to 13 years, 25% (25,400 visits) were related to organized team sports (football, hockey, soccer, baseball, and basketball) and 75% (76,600 visits) with leisure and individual sports (bicycling, skiing, equestrian, sledding, playground).[12]

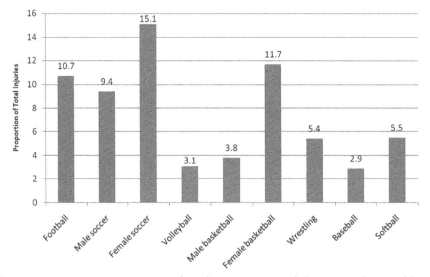

Fig. 1. Concussions as a percentage of total injuries sustained. (*From* Gessel LM, Fields SK, Collins CL, et al. Concussions among United States high school and collegiate athletes. J Athl Train 2007;42(4):500; with permission.)

SELECTED YOUTH SPORTS

All numbers mentioned later are for the United States (unless otherwise specified).

Concussion incidence studies are often published using a rate of injury per occurrence per 1000 athletic exposures (AE). AE are defined as an athletes' participation in a single practice or competition. To give a rough estimate, 15 athletes playing in a game or practicing 5 days per week for 3 months (13 weeks) gives 975 AE. Thus, a rate of 0.5 injuries per 1000 AE requires an injury to 1 out of 30 athletes playing games or practicing for about 13 weeks. **Table 1** shows the number of concussions per 1000 AE in high school based on sport, gender, and overall.

Baseball and Softball

Baseball and softball are 2 of the most popular sports in the United States involving millions of athletes.[13-15] Many participants are youth recreational athletes, with an estimated 1.7 million athletes per year.[16] Approximately 450,000 boys participate in high school baseball, and 313,000 girls participate in high school softball, annually.[17]

Overall, there has been a decrease in the number of baseball- and softball-related injuries in the past few decades but an increase in the severity of injuries, especially involving the head and face region. Powell and Barber-Foss'[18,19] studies of injury patterns in high school sports from 1996 to 1997 reported 1.5 to 2.8 baseball-related injuries per 1000 AE and 1.6 to 3.5 softball-related injures per 1000 AE. The investigators reported 0.23 concussions per season for every 100 athletes. During the 2005 to 2006 season, Rechel and colleagues'[20] study of high school sports reported 1.77 baseball-related injuries per 1000 AE during games and 0.87 injuries per 1000 AE during practice. Of these injuries, there were 0.08 concussions per 1000 AE during games and 0.03 concussions per 1000 AE during practices. The investigators reported 1.79 softball-related injuries during games and 0.79 injuries per 1000 AE during practices. Of these injuries, there were 0.04 concussions per 1000 AE during games and 0.09 concussions per 1000 AE during practices. Collins and Comstock[15] analyzed high school baseball injury rates (2005–2007), reporting an overall injury rate of 1.26 injuries per 1000 AE, with a higher injury rate during competition (1.89 per

Table 1
Concussion rates in high school sports by sport and gender

Sport	Gessel et al,[8] 2007 Concussion Rate (per 1000 AE)	Lincoln et al,[24] 2011 Concussion Rate (per 1000 AE)
Baseball	0.05	0.06
Softball	0.07	0.11
Boys' Basketball	0.07	0.1
Girls' Basketball	0.21	0.16
Boys' Soccer	0.22	0.17
Girls' Soccer	0.36	0.35
Football	0.47	0.6
Wrestling	0.18	0.17
All Boys	NR	0.34
All Girls	NR	0.13
All Athletes	NR	0.24

Abbreviation: NR, not reported.

athlete practices) versus practice (0.85 per athlete practices). Among all body regions, head and face injuries accounted for 12.3% of all injuries. Of these head and face injuries, concussions (28.7%) occurred as frequently as fractures (28.7%). Concussion involved only 3.5% of the overall diagnoses but represented an injury rate of 0.11 injuries per 1000 AE. Gessel's[8] study of 100 US high schools during the 2005 to 2006 season reported similar concussion rates between baseball (0.07 per 1000 AE) and softball (0.05 per 1000 AE) but a greater portion of total injuries in softball (5.5%) than baseball players (2.9%).

The most common mechanisms of injury relating to concussions in baseball or softball occurred from contact between a player and a ball, bat, or base. Collins'[15] study of high school baseball players reports that concussions were more likely to occur from being hit by a batted ball (8%) than other mechanisms of injury (2.9%), although this was not statistically significant. Gessel and colleagues'[8] study of high school athletes noted that baseball players compared with softball players were more likely to experience a concussion from contact with a ball (91.4% vs 59.1%) and to be associated with being hit by a pitch (50.6% vs 6.9%). Injuries varied depending on the specific player positions, with head and face injuries most likely to occur in batters (19.7%), outfielders (16.8%), and infielders (15%). Concussions were slightly higher in batters (4.6%) and outfielders (4.1%) than in catchers (3.6%), infielders (3.5%), and pitchers (3.3%). Base runners were the least likely to experience any of the various injuries.

Studies of baseball and softball players have revealed interesting findings regarding the rate of symptom recovery and return to play. Symptom resolution (ie, <6 days) seems to occur earlier in softball players than in baseball players (68.8% vs 64.2%; injury). However, a greater percentage of baseball players return to play within 6 days than softball players (52.9% vs 15.5%; injury). Fortunately, in both baseball players and softball players, more than 90% return to play within 10 to 21 days.[8]

Severe and catastrophic youth baseball-related injuries are quite rare.[13,21,22] Lawson and colleagues'[21] study of baseball-related injuries in children presenting to the EDs in the United States from 1994 to 2006 reported that 5.8% of all injuries were caused by concussions and closed head injuries. Only 3 cases were identified to be fatal injuries over the study period. The most common mechanism of injury was being struck by a baseball (46%) or being hit by the bat (24.9%). Athletes aged 12 to 17 years had the highest injury rate (19.8 per 1000 athletes) compared with younger athletes aged 6 to 11 years (12.1 per 1000 athletes). Boden and colleagues'[13] study of the incidence of catastrophic baseball-related injuries between 1981 and 2002 reported 33 catastrophic injuries in high school athletes, with 65% relating to severe head injuries. The overall direct catastrophic injury rate was 0.37 per 100,000 high school baseball players. The most common mechanism of injury was between a player and a ball involving a pitcher being struck in the head by a batted ball (56%) compared with a fielder (8%) or a batter (4%) being hit by a pitched ball. In most of these cases involving pitchers, the batter was using an aluminum bat.

Basketball

Basketball is the most popular female high school sport, with 448,450 athletes in 2008, and the second most popular male high school sport, with 552,935 athletes.[23]

A 2006 study showed that girls had a higher rate of concussion (0.21 concussions per 1000 AE) than boys (0.07 concussions per 1000 AE).[8] The difference is found almost exclusively in games. Both boys and girls have a rate of 0.06 concussions per 1000 AE in practice. In games, the concussion rate in boys roughly doubles to

0.11, whereas in girls the concussion rate increases 10-fold to 0.60. The same study reported concussions representing 11.7% of total injuries in girls and only 3.8% in boys. Girls were most likely to suffer injury while defending another player and with ball handling/dribbling. Boys were more likely to suffer head injury while chasing down loose balls and rebounding and due to contact with the playing surface.

An 11-year study from 1997 to 2008 showed boys' basketball with a rate of 0.10 concussions per 1000 AE and girls' basketball with a higher rate of 0.16. The concussion rate increased for both boys and girls over the evaluation period.[24]

Catastrophic head injury in basketball

From 1982 to 1999, there was 1 reported fatality in high school basketball, 0 injuries resulting in permanent disability, and 4 serious head injuries that resolved without permanent sequelae.[25]

Cheerleading

There is an increase in participation in cheerleading, with Daneshvar and colleagues[17] reporting that the number of athletes has increased 18% overall since 1990. At present, there are an estimated 3.5 million participants within the United States.[17] This includes 22,900 estimated participants (in 2002) between the ages of 5 and 18 years.[26] Shields and Smith[26] report that a 110% increase in participation has been seen for this age group since 1990 (10,900 participants compared with 22,900 participants in 2002). The investigators report that one of the leading causes in participant increase is also responsible for the rising prevalence of concussion: the maneuvers performed by the teams have become more difficult and more gymnasticslike. Daneshvar and colleagues[17] indicate a significant increase in injury between 1980 and 2007, with 4954 ED visits in 1980 jumping to 26,786 ED visits in 2007. The investigators cite tumbling rings, pyramids, lifts, catches, and tosses as moves that have increased injury. The flier is particularly at risk as are those in the bottom quintile for body mass index.[3,17]

Apart from the gymnastics element, concussion may also be the result of collisions with other cheerleaders.[27] Cheerleading is one of the only sports to show a higher rate of concussion in practice than games (11.32 concussions per 1000 AE vs 3.38 concussions per 1000 AE).[3] Daneshvar and colleagues[17] found supporting evidence, reporting 82% of injury to occur during practice rather than game exposures. Schultz and colleagues[2] found a rate of 9.36 head injuries per 1000 AE, whereas Shields and colleagues[27] found a head injury rate of 5.7% among high school participants.

Football

In 2008, there were 1,100,000 high school football athletes and approximately 400,000 junior high school and junior football athletes.[23] Football consistently shows the highest rate of concussion for all youth sports. A 3-year prospective study (1995–1997) found an incidence of 5.1% per season. About 14.7% of these players suffered a second concussion during the same season.[28]

Data from a year-long study in 2006 showed a rate of 0.47 per 1000 AE. On defense, linebackers were shown to have the highest rate of concussion (40.9%). On offense, no significant difference was noted by position. The highest proportion of concussion occurs during running plays and resulted from contact with another player. Concussions were 7 times more likely to happen in games than practice (1.55 vs 0.21 per 1000 AE).[8] A 2011 study showed that high school football reported a concussion rate of 0.60 per 1000 AE over an 11-year period from 1997 to 2008. The study also found an increase in concussion rate of 8% per year.[24]

A 2004 retrospective survey study of concussion found that many high school football players underreported concussion. The study estimated that 15% of high school players suffered a concussion each season and 47.2% did not report having a concussion.[29]

Catastrophic head injuries

Over a 13-year period (1989–2002), there were 92 catastrophic head injuries associated with high school football. During this same period, there were only 2 incidents at the college level. This averages to 7.23 events per year in high school and college sports. Of the total 94 head injuries, there were 8 (8.9%) fatalities, 46 injuries (51.1%) that left permanent neurologic damage and, 36 injuries (40%) that recovered completely. Of the patients whose past history was obtainable, 59.3% reported having a previous head injury before the day of the catastrophic event, and 38.9% of the respondents reported playing with residual neurologic symptoms from a previous head injury.[30] High school sports in 2008 were associated with 43 direct catastrophic injuries, and all were associated with football. These injuries included 7 fatalities, 20 injuries that resulted in permanent disability, and 16 injuries that were considered serious but showed complete recovery. Of the 7 fatalities, 5 were related to head injury. Listed causes of death included subdural hematoma, brain injury, and second impact syndrome. This was the highest rate of injury since data collection began in 1982.[31]

Ice Hockey

Ice hockey has an estimated 530,000 players in the United States, a number that includes 370,458 youth participants.[32] Daneshvar and colleagues[17] report that 27,800 men and 2800 women compete in the sport each year. Checking, hit contact allowed in ice hockey, begins at very young ages, sometimes as early as 9 years, and is often cited for the high volume of injuries as well as the elevated rate of concussions observed when compared with other sports. It is speculated that the youth are not given proper instructions on body checking and therefore are more likely to injure other players.[32]

Hostetler and colleagues[32] found that traumatic brain injury (TBI) rates decreased with age, which may be because of better playing techniques. Daneshvar and colleagues,[17] however, reported the opposite, indicating in their article that recent studies have shown that players in the Bantam (aged 13–14 years) and Pee Wee (aged 12–13 years) groups had an increased risk of concussion compared with the Atom (aged 9–10 years) group. The investigators suggest the start of body checking as the reason for the increase in concussion observation. In players younger than 18 years, Hostetler and colleagues[32] found that TBI accounted for 14.1% of all ice hockey–related injuries, whereas Hagel and colleagues[33] found concussion to account for 6.4% of injuries at the Atom (aged 10–11 years) level and 12.6% at the Pee Wee (aged 12–13 years) level. Daneshvar and colleagues[17] reported that concussions account for 6.3% of injuries occurring during practice exposures, and 10.3% of injuries during the game. Echlin and colleagues[34] report an overall incidence of 21.52 concussions per 1000 AE. Johnson[35] indicated that 25.3% of youth players received at least 1 concussion during the course of 1 season. Echlin and colleagues[34] reported that after return to play from a concussion, 97% of recurrence of injury occurs within 10 days of the initial injury and 75% occur within 7 days. This increased susceptibility suggests that players may be returning to play too quickly.

Previous studies suggest that eliminating body checking from youth leagues may be the best way to prevent head injuries in this athlete population. Echlin and colleagues[34] report that 24% of concussions followed a fight and that most concussions followed some form of a hit to the head. Preventing this hit may also provide a way to decrease concussion incidence. In Canada, Johnson[35] indicates that the only junior league that continues to see an increase in players is in Quebec because they do not allow body checking until the Bantam level (ages, 14–15 years). The rest of the country is experiencing a decrease in participation. Hagel and colleagues[33] and Daneshvar and colleagues[17] both report that leagues that permit body checking are associated with a significantly higher occurrence of concussion.

Lacrosse

Lacrosse is one of the fastest growing sports in the United States. Most collegiate teams are located in the East Coast region, but there has been an expansion of teams toward the West Coast region. It is estimated that 33,000 male and 22,000 female high school athletes participate in lacrosse any given year. Despite the increasing level of participation, there are very few studies assessing the impact of concussions in lacrosse athletes at the high school level.[14,17]

The few studies of high school lacrosse athletes suggest a greater number of concussions in boys versus girls. Lincoln and colleagues[36] studied head and neck injuries in 507,000 high school lacrosse athletes (both boys and girls) over 4 seasons (2000–2003). Concussions represented a higher percentage of injuries among boys (73%) than among girls (40%). Concussion rates were 0.28 per 1000 AE for boys versus 0.21 per 1000 AE for girls. These findings were similar to concussion rates in collegiate athletes (0.26 per 1000 AE in men [95% confidence interval (CI) 5, 0.23–0.39]; 0.25 per 1000 AE in women [95% CI 5, 0.22–0.28]) from 1988 through 2004.[37,38] In a similar study, Lincoln[24] examined the incidence and relative risk of concussions in 12 high school boys' and girls' sports from 1997 to 2008. Concussions represented 9.2% (boys) and 4.3% (girls) of all injuries during the study period. Concussion rates were 0.3 per 1000 AE (CI 5.5, 4.9–6.3) for boys and 0.20 per 1000 AE (CI 3.5, 2.9–4.2) for girls. The investigators reported a mean annual increase in concussions per year of 17% and 14% for boys and girls, respectively. The main injury mechanism for boys was player-to-player contact, whereas for girls it was stick or ball contact. These findings differed from collegiate lacrosse, in which 78.4% of men's concussions resulted from a collision with another person, whereas 10.4% resulted from collision with a stick.[37] More than half the time, the concussions in female collegiate lacrosse players resulted from contact with a stick.[38] The difference in mechanisms of injury between boys and girls most likely reflects differences in the games relating to protective equipment (boys use helmets, whereas girls do not) rules and level of contact permitted (greater in boys). There have been no reported catastrophic injuries relating to concussions in high school lacrosse players over the past 2 decades.[14]

Soccer

Participation in soccer has grown over the past few decades. In the United States, an estimated 13 to 15 million youth athletes participate in soccer at the recreational to elite levels. Almost 3.2 million participate in the US Youth Soccer Association, representing athletes younger than 19 years.[17,40] From 2009 to 2010, more than 745,000 boys and girls participated in high school soccer, making it the fifth most popular sport in the United States.[23] However, with increased participation has come a potential increase in the number of concussions.

Overall, there seems to be an increase in the number of concussions reported by soccer athletes over the past few decades. However, there are conflicting data regarding the differences in the rate of concussions between young boy and girl soccer athletes. An earlier study from 1990 to 2003 revealed an estimated 1.9% of pediatric (ages, 2–18 years) soccer-related injuries presenting to the ED were caused by concussions.[39] A 2005 to 2006 study of US high school soccer athletes revealed an overall rate of 0.22 concussions per 1000 AE in boys compared with 0.36 concussions per 1000 AE in girls.[8] Both were more likely to sustain a concussion during games (girls, 0.97 per 1000 AE; boys, 0.59 per 1000 AE) than practices (girls, 0.09 per 1000 AE; boys, 0.04 per 1000 AE). A study of high school soccer athletes from 2005 to 2007 revealed that boys and girls sustained a similar rate of concussions (9.3% and 12.2%, respectively) (injury proportion ratio [IPR], 1.31; 95% CI, 0.91–1.88) but at a higher rate than what was previously reported.[42] Similar to other studies, the investigators did report a greater rate of concussions occurring during games versus practices (IPR, 3.25; 95% CI, 1.99–5.31). A study of recurrent injuries in high school soccer athletes revealed a similar rate of concussions in boys versus girls (9.2% vs 10.6%) but a higher reinjury rate in girls than in boys (19.1% vs 13.8%).[41] Whether girls truly have a higher risk of sustaining a concussion is not exactly clear. Factors contributing to the perceived increased rate could include a greater awareness of concussions or greater propensity to report concussive symptoms.

The most common mechanisms of injury relating to concussions in soccer players involve head-to-head collisions, contact with the ground, or contact with the ball. Several studies have shown that soccer players were most likely to sustain a concussion from a head-to-head collision while attempting to head the ball.[8,42,43] In a study by Gessel and colleagues,[8] boys were more likely than girls to experience concussion via this mechanism (40.5% in boys vs 36.7% in girls [IPR, 1.46; 95% CI, 1.45–1.48; P<.01]). Girls were more likely to sustain a concussion from contact with the ground (22.6% vs 6.0% [IPR, 3.77; 95% CI, 3.56–4.00; P<.01]) and contact with the soccer ball (18.3% vs 8.2% [IPR, 3.68; 95% CI, 3.45–3.92; P<.01]). Similarly, Yard's[42] study reported that 71.8% of athletes experienced concussions from a head-to-head collision. Athletes were less likely to sustain a concussion from contact with the ground (16.1%) or contact with the ball only (7%). The investigators noted that illegal activity contributed to 25.3% of concussions (IPR, 1.92; 95% CI, 1.16–3.16) compared with injuries caused by legal activities. Injuries were more likely to occur to goalkeepers (21.7%) than to players in other positions (11.1%) (IPR, 1.96; 95% CI, 1.92–2.00; P<.01).[8]

Studies of time loss and return to play reveal that most concussions in soccer players among high school athletes require several days to a couple of weeks to resolve.[9,43] A recent study of high school athletes suggests that 46.1% require approximately 7 to 21 days to recover, followed by 38.9% requiring less than 7 days to recover.[43] Severe injuries were much less common, with 11% of boys and 7.4% of girls experiencing a concussion lasting longer than 3 weeks. In this study, 7.3% of concussions were season ending. Despite several published return-to-play guidelines, Yard and Comstock[7] revealed noncompliance with the Prague return-to-play guidelines ranging from 15% to 19% for boy and girl high school soccer players.

Despite the potential for head-to-head collisions in youth soccer, catastrophic events are exceedingly rare. Longitudinal studies have reported 17 to 28 catastrophic head and neck injuries from participation in youth soccer between 1982 and 2008.[14,31] Reported direct injuries per 100,000 athletes were 0.1 (fatal), 0.03 (permanent neurologic deficits), and 0.08 (serious injury with complete recovery) for youth boys and 0 (fatal), 0.02 (permanent neurologic deficits), and 0.02 (serious injury with complete recovery) for youth girls. A good number of these injuries related to goal posts falling onto the youth soccer athlete. Several recommendations including keeping soccer goals anchored, never allowing children to hang or climb soccer goals, removing the soccer goals when not in use, and periodic maintenance have led to a significant decrease in these fatalities.

Wrestling

A total of 259,688 boys were involved in wrestling in high school in 2008. Female wrestling is also on the increase, with approximately 1700 female athletes.[17,23]

A 2006 study showed a concussion rate of 0.18 concussions per 1000 AE with 3 times the rate in competition than practice (0.32 and 0.13, respectively).[8] Over 11 years, Lincoln and colleagues[24] found a similar rate of 0.17. This rate was increasing over time at a rate of 27% per year.

Takedowns were the most common maneuver or activity associated with concussion (42.6%). Contact with another person (60.1%) was the major cause of concussion as opposed to contact with the playing surface (26.9%).[7] Catastrophic head injury is very low; from 1982 to 1999, there were 1 fatality in high school wrestling and no injuries with permanent disability.[25]

REFERENCES

1. Thurman DJ, Branche CM, Sniezek JE. The epidemiology of sports related traumatic brain injuries in the United States: recent developments. J Head Trauma Rehabil 1998;13(2):1–8.
2. Schultz MR, Marshall SW, Mueller FO, et al. Incidence and risk factors for concussion in high school athletes, North Carolina, 1996-1999. Am J Epidemiol 2004; 160(10):933–44.
3. Collins MW, Iverson GL, Lovell MR, et al. On-field predictors of neuropsychological and symptom deficit following sports-related concussion. Clin J Sport Med 2003;13(4):222–9.
4. Langlois JA, Rutland-Brown W, Wald MM. The epidemiology and impact of traumatic brain injury: a brief overview. J Head Trauma Rehabil 2006;21(5): 375–8.
5. Government Accountability Office. Concussion in high school sports. Available at: http://www.gao.gov/new.items/d10569t.pdf. Accessed February 24, 2011.
6. Grady MF. Concussion in the adolescent athlete. Curr Probl Pediatr Adolesc Health Care 2010;40(7):154–69.
7. Yard EE, Comstock RD. Compliance with return to play guidelines following concussion in US high school athletes, 2005–2008. Brain Inj 2009;23(11):888–98.
8. Gessel LM, Fields SK, Collins CL, et al. Concussions among United States high school and collegiate athletes. J Athl Train 2007;42(4):495–503.
9. Field M, Collins MW, Lovell MR, et al. Does age play a role in recovery from sports-related concussion? A comparison of high school and collegiate athletes. J Pediatr 2003;142(5):546–53.
10. McClincy MP, Lovell MR, Pardini J, et al. Recovery from sports concussion in high school and collegiate athletes. Brain Inj 2006;20(1):33–9.
11. Fommer LJ, Gurka KK, Cross KM, et al. Sex differences in concussion symptoms of high school athletes. J Athl Train 2011;46(1):76–84.
12. Bakhos LL, Lockhart GR, Myers R, et al. Emergency department visits for concussion in young child athletes. Pediatrics 2010;126:e550–6.
13. Boden BP, Tacchetti R, Mueller FO. Catastrophic injuries in high school and college baseball players. Am J Sports Med 2004;32(5):1189–96.
14. Cantu RC, Mueller FO. The prevention of catastrophic head and spine injuries in high school and college sports. Br J Sports Med 2009;43(13):981–6.

15. Collins CL, Comstock RD. Epidemiological features of high school baseball injuries in the United States, 2005-2007. Pediatrics 2008;121(6):1181-7.
16. Mueller FO, Marshall SW, Kirby DO. Injuries in little league baseball from 1987 though 1996. Phys Sportsmed 2001;29(7):41-8.
17. Daneshvar DH, Nowinski CJ, McKee AC, et al. The epidemiology of sport-related concussion. Clin Sports Med 2011;30(1):1-17, vii.
18. Powell JW, Barber-Foss KD. Injury patterns in selected high school sports: a review of the 1995-1997 seasons. J Athl Train 1999;34(3):277-84.
19. Powell JW, Barber-Foss KD. Sex-related injury patterns among selected high school sports. Am J Sports Med 2000;28(3):385-91.
20. Rechel JA, Yard EE, Comstock RD. An epidemiologic comparison of high school sports injuries sustained in practice and competition. J Athl Train 2008;43(2): 197-204.
21. Lawson BR, Comstock RD, Smith GA. Baseball-related injuries to children treated in hospital emergency departments in the United States, 1994-2006. Pediatrics 2009;123(6):e1028-34.
22. Huffman EA, Yard EE, Fields SK, et al. Epidemiology of rare injuries and conditions among United States high school athletes during the 2005-2006 and 2006-2007 school years. J Athl Train 2008;43(6):624-30.
23. National Federation of High Schools. 2009–10 High School Athletics Participation Study. Available at: http://www.nfhs.org/search.aspx?searchtext=soccer%20 participation. Accessed February 4, 2011.
24. Lincoln AE, Caswell SV, Almquist JL, et al. Trends in concussion in high school sports: a prospective 11-year study. Am J Sports Med 2011;39(5):958-63.
25. Mueller FO. Catastrophic head injuries in high school and collegiate sports. J Athl Train 2001;36(3):312-5.
26. Shields BJ, Smith GA. Cheerleading-related injuries in the United States: a prospective surveillance study. J Athl Train 2009;44(6):567-77.
27. Shields BJ, Soledad SA, Smith GA. Epidemiology of cheerleading stunt-related injuries in the United States. J Athl Train 2009;44(6):586-94.
28. Guskiewicz KM, Weaver NL, Padua DA, et al. Epidemiology of concussion in collegiate and high school football players. Am J Sports Med 2000;28(5):643-50.
29. McCrea M, Hammeke T, Olsen G, et al. Unreported concussion in high school football players. Clin J Sport Med 2004;14(1):13-7.
30. Boden BP, Tacchetti RL, Cantu RC, et al. Catastrophic head injuries in high school and college football players. AM J Sports Med 2007;35(7):1075-81.
31. Mueller FO, Cantu RC. Catastrophic Sports Injury Research Twenty-Sixth Annual Report Fall 1982—Spring 2008. Available at: http://www.unc.edu/depts/nccsi. Accessed March 1, 2011.
32. Hostetler SG, Xiang H, Smith GA. Characteristics of ice hockey-related injuries treated in US emergency departments, 2001-2002. Pediatrics 2004;114:e661-6.
33. Hagel BE, Marko J, Dryden D, et al. Effect of bodychecking on injury rates among minor ice hockey players. Can Med Assoc J 2006;175(2):155-60.
34. Echlin PS, Tator CH, Cusimano MD, et al. A prospective study of physician-observed concussions during junior ice hockey: implications for incidence rates. Neurosurg Focus 2010;29(5):1-10.
35. Johnson LSM. Concussion in youth ice hockey: it's time to break the cycle. Can Med Assoc J 2011;183(8):921-4.
36. Lincoln AE, Hinton RY, Almquist JL, et al. Head, face, and eye injuries in scholastic and collegiate lacrosse: a 4-year prospective study. Am J Sports Med 2007;35(2):207-15.

37. Dick R, Romani WA, Agel J, et al. Descriptive epidemiology of collegiate men's lacrosse injuries: national collegiate athletic association injury surveillance system, 1988–1989 through 2003–2004. J Athl Train 2007;42(2):255–61.
38. Dick R, Lincoln AE, Agel J, et al. Descriptive epidemiology of collegiate women's lacrosse injuries: National Collegiate Athletic Association Injury Surveillance System, 1988–1989 through 2003–2004. J Athl Train 2007;42(2):262–9.
39. Leininger RE, Knox CL, Comstock RD. Epidemiology of 1.6 million pediatric soccer-related injuries presenting to US emergency departments from 1990 to 2003. Am J Sports Med 2007;35:288–93.
40. Koutures CG, Gregory AJ. Injuries in youth soccer. Pediatrics 2010;125(2):410–4.
41. Swenson DM, Yard EE, Fields SK, et al. Patterns of recurrent injuries among US high school athletes, 2005-2008. Am J Sports Med 2009;37(8):1586–93.
42. Yard EE, Schroeder MJ, Fields SK, et al. The epidemiology of United States high school soccer injuries, 2005-2007. Am J Sports Med 2008;36(10):1930–7.
43. Junge A, Cheung K, Edwards T, et al. Injuries in youth amateur soccer and rugby players—comparison of incidence and characteristics. Br J Sports Med 2004; 38(2):168–72.

The Pathophysiology of Concussions in Youth

Daniel W. Shrey, MD[a],*, Grace S. Griesbach, PhD[b],
Christopher C. Giza, MD[a,b]

KEYWORDS

- Traumatic brain injury • Metabolic cascade • Activation
- Plasticity • Pediatrics

Mild traumatic brain injury (TBI) or concussion is estimated to occur in millions of persons annually in the United States alone. The peak ages for these injuries are in adolescence and young adulthood, and sport-related concussions are particularly common among young persons.[1] Although generally these injuries are self-limited, the consequences of even transient pathophysiologic dysfunction must be carefully considered in the context of a developing or immature brain, as must the potential for an accumulation of damage with repeated exposure over a long period. This article reviews the underlying neurometabolic cascade of concussion, with emphasis on the young brain in terms of acute pathophysiology, vulnerability, alterations in plasticity, axonal injury, and risk for chronic cumulative deficits.

ACUTE METABOLIC CASCADE
Glutamate Release and Ionic Disequilibrium

The postconcussive metabolic cascade has been well studied and character-ized, both in animal models and in humans. As a result of mechanical trauma, neuronal cell membranes and axons undergo disruptive stretching, leading to temporary ionic disequilibrium.[2] As a result, levels of extracellular potassium

This work was supported by: NS27544, NS057420, NS06190, the Child Neurology Foundation/ Winokur Family Foundation, the Today's and Tomorrow's Children Fund, and the UCLA Brain Injury Research Center.

The authors have nothing to disclose.

[a] Division of Pediatric Neurology, Department of Pediatrics, David Geffen School of Medicine at UCLA, Mattel Children's Hospital, UCLA, Room 22-474 MDCC, 10833 Le Conte Boulevard, Los Angeles, CA 90095, USA

[b] Department of Neurosurgery, UCLA Brain Injury Research Center, Semel Institute, David Geffen School of Medicine at UCLA, PO Box 957039, 10833 Le Conte Avenue, Los Angeles, CA 90095-7039, USA

* Corresponding author.

E-mail address: dshrey@mednet.ucla.edu

Phys Med Rehabil Clin N Am 22 (2011) 577–602
doi:10.1016/j.pmr.2011.08.002
1047-9651/11/$ – see front matter © 2011 Elsevier Inc. All rights reserved.

increase drastically, and indiscriminate glutamate release occurs.[3] Glutamate release activates N-methyl-D-aspartate receptors, which leads to accumulation of intracellular calcium,[4–6] causing mitochondrial respiration dysfunction, protease activation, and often initiating apoptosis.[7,8] Increased glutamate levels were also found to be significantly correlated with derangements in lactate, potassium, brain tissue pH, and brain tissue CO_2 levels in human studies.[9] In addition, sodium channel upregulation, fueled by adenosine triphosphatase proteins depending on glucose for energy, is observed after axonal stretch injuries.[10]

Energy Crisis and Mitochondrial Dysfunction

In combination, the cellular response to the ionic shifts and the downstream effects of the neurotransmitter release mentioned earlier lead to an acute energy crisis. This crisis occurs when, to restore ionic equilibrium, adenosine triphosphate (ATP)-dependent sodium-potassium ion transporter pump activity increases, which augments local cerebral glucose demand.[11] Further metabolic demand is incurred by ATP-dependent sodium channel upregulation. This demand occurs in the face of mitochondrial dysfunction, leading cells to primarily use glycolytic pathways instead of aerobic metabolism for energy, and causing extracellular lactate accumulation as a byproduct.[12] This acidosis, caused by hyperglycolysis, has been shown to worsen membrane permeability, ionic disequilibrium, and cerebral edema.[13]

Some evidence shows that the lactate produced by this process may eventually be used as a source of energy by the neurons once mitochondrial oxidative respiration normalizes; 1 study showed that in moderate to severe TBI the incidence of abnormally high levels of lactate uptake was seen in 28% of patients.[14] The same study showed that patients showing a higher rate of brain lactate uptake relative to arterial lactate levels tended to have more favorable outcomes compared with others with lower relative lactate uptake.

Alterations in Cerebral Blood Flow

Cerebral blood flow (CBF) changes after severe TBI have also been well studied. A triphasic response to severe TBI has been characterized, specifically showing hypoperfusion on postinjury day 0, hyperperfusion on postinjury days 1 to 3, and vasospasm on postinjury days 4 to 15.[15] Regarding mild TBI, some studies have shown that CBF decreases immediately after the insult, and the amount of time it remains decreased seems to depend on the severity of the injury.[16,17] However, other studies show no significant differences in CBF after mild TBI in patients more than 30 years of age.[18] In pediatric studies, CBF has been seen to increase during the first day after mild TBI, followed by decreased CBF for many days after.[19,20] Data comparing CBF in pediatric patients with TBI have shown impaired autoregulation in 42% of moderate and severe and 17% of mild injuries.[21] In severe TBI, impaired autoregulation was associated with worsened long-term outcomes.[22]

VULNERABILITY TO SECOND INJURY AND SECOND IMPACT SYNDROME

Postconcussive physiologic changes have been shown to increase the vulnerability of the brain to further injury, particularly in cases in which a second concussive injury is sustained within days of the first. This phenomenon can lead to more severe and permanent deficits. Numerous studies, both in animal models and in humans, support the concept of postconcussive vulnerability, prompting the development of many sets of return-to-play guidelines.[23–28] Research has shown that having a history of concussion increases an individual's probability of having a future concussion as well as prolonging the duration of significantly abnormal cognitive functioning.[29] These data support increased awareness of postconcussive vulnerability and suggest adherence to return-to-play guidelines may be helpful.

In addition, an extreme entity termed second impact syndrome has been postulated, in which an individual experiencing a second mild TBI within days of the first can experience diffuse cerebral swelling and catastrophic deterioration.[30,31] Second impact syndrome remains somewhat controversial in definition and explanation,[27,31–33] with most of the literature addressing its existence being case reports. The pathophysiology of second impact syndrome is believed to result from the combined effects of increased intracranial blood volume (secondary to loss of CBF autoregulation) and posttraumatic catecholamine release, leading to catastrophic cerebral edema, generally in the absence of major hematomas or other space-occupying lesions.[33–35] McCrory and Berkovic[32] proposed diagnostic criteria in 1998 to facilitate more consistent analysis of potential cases of second impact syndrome, as well as to diminish the bias involved in case reporting. After applying these criteria, many of the previously reported cases of second impact syndrome were found to fall short of diagnosis. Nonetheless, there is recognition of a syndrome of malignant cerebral edema after mild TBI, and multiple reviews and case series of second impact syndrome have been published.[33,36,37] A similar syndrome has been described in individuals harboring a calcium channel mutation (CACNA1A) associated with familial hemiplegic migraine.[38]

Experimental

Numerous basic science studies have investigated the consequences of sustaining 2 closely timed brain injuries compared with a single insult, characterizing the effects on brain damage and cognitive deficits.[23–26,39] As described earlier, neurons undergo significant changes in metabolism, blood flow, and energy usage after a single TBI. These changes in cellular function contribute to transient dysfunction after injury, but in mild TBI, cellular recovery eventually occurs, typically with minimal anatomic changes/damage.[40] Metabolic derangements in N-acetylaspartate°(NAA), ATP, and ATP/adenosine diphosphate ratios after concussive brain injuries in rats have been studied. Results showed that 2 concussive injuries separated by 3 days showed derangements significantly worse than either a single injury or 2 injuries with 5 days separation.[41] A more recent study by Vagnozzi and colleagues,[25] who measured other biochemical markers of mitochondrial dysfunction in rats sustaining 2 mild TBIs, showed comparable findings. Another notable result was that a second impact at 5 days after the first showed metabolic changes equivalent to the first impact but not more severe. Sustained oxidative and nitrosative stresses have also been shown to follow a similar pattern, with peak derangements noted with a second impact occurring 3 days after the first.[24]

These results corroborated those of an earlier study from 2005 by Longhi and colleagues,[39] who compared mice with 1 concussive event or 2 concussive events 1, 3, 5, or 7 days apart with control mice that underwent sham injuries. This study showed significant cognitive deficits in mice concussed twice at intervals of 3 and 5 days but not in those concussed only once, or concussed twice but at 1-day or 7-day intervals. This finding supports the notion of a defined interval after an initial insult during which there is increased propensity for greater deficits should a second trauma occur. This study also showed a significantly increased degree of traumatic axonal injury mice sustaining a second injury 3 days after the first injury when compared with mice with only a single concussion.

Other studies have focused on histologic and cognitive changes after mild TBI.[26,42] It has been shown that experimental closed head injury in juvenile rats can cause cognitive deficits in the absence of gross pathology or high mortality. However, a second injury performed 1 day after the first caused increased memory impairment as well as neuropathologic changes of increased axonal injury and astrocytic reactivity.[26] This study is also the only experimental study of repeated mild TBI conducted in immature animals, thus targeting the age group at highest risk for such injuries in humans. Another study showed impairment in the Morris water maze task after 3 sequential concussive head traumas causing transient loss of consciousness, but these injuries also caused contracoup neuropathologic changes compared with non-concussed controls.[42]

Human Studies

Magnetic resonance spectroscopy (MRS) has been used to assess cellular changes after sustaining TBI.[23,43,44] Vagnozzi and colleagues,[23] using voxels in the white matter of the bilateral frontal lobes immediately adjacent to the cortical-subcortical junction, assessed the ratio of NAA to creatine (Cr) specifically in athletes after concussion. Concussed athletes showed a decrease (−18.5%) in the NAA/Cr ratio on postinjury day 3 compared with age-matched, nonconcussed controls (1.80 ± 0.04 vs 2.15 ± 0.1; $P<.001$), with return to normal values by 30 days after concussion. A second concussive event prolonged the time of NAA/Cr normalization by 15 days, with NAA/Cr values remaining significantly less than normal (1.82 ± 0.1) at 30 days, and return to normalcy noted only at 45 days (2.07 ± 0.1).[23]

Data described in these studies, coupled with the lack of consensus regarding management of concussion based on clinical evaluation alone, support supplementing clinical assessment by using biomarkers. This strategy would add more objectivity and allow for better-defined return-to-play recommendations. The necessity of including such data in gauging severity of TBI and recovery stems from showing that an absence of clinical signs or symptoms does not always coincide with completed brain metabolic recovery. Conversely, it is still unclear whether metabolic alterations in the absence of measurable clinical impairment indicate an underlying vulnerable state. A potentially valuable approach might be to identify clinical measures that closely reflect the underlying metabolic state in a subset of athletes, because it is currently impractical to propose routine use of MRS for all concussions. Ideally, the approach to management of a concussed individual would then involve monitoring of clinical status in all and metabolic biomarkers in a selected subset of athletes.

IMPAIRED/ABNORMAL ACTIVATION AFTER TBI
Experimental

Experimental brain injury models have indicated that brain activation is altered for several weeks after TBI. Changes in excitability and circuit function have not only been observed in more severe brain injury but also after mild TBI.[45,46] Anatomic changes after trauma along with subtle changes in neuronal properties influence neuronal excitability. These postinjury changes in brain activation have an array of consequences ranging from alterations in synaptic plasticity,[46] axonal sprouting[47] and excitatory-inhibitory imbalance.[48] These underlying physiologic changes may then manifest phenotypically as cognitive impairments or increased risk of seizures/epilepsy.[49]

After a brain injury, metabolic alterations occur that result in subacute hypometabolism. The duration of this metabolic disturbance is believed to be associated with the severity of the injury.[50] These metabolic changes are likely to influence brain activation.[6,51–53] Changes in excitability also have an effect on calcium regulation and thus on molecular markers of plasticity such as neurotrophins. Animal research indicates that neurotrophin expression, such as brain-derived neurotrophic factor (BDNF), is regulated by neural activity.[54,55] In turn, alterations in BDNF also influence brain activation given its role on synaptic facilitation[56] and neurotransmitter release enhancement.[57–59] For example, BDNF levels normally increase in response to exercise[60]; however, this is not observed if exercise occurs during the first days after a fluid-percussion injury (FPI).[61] Among these lines, cortical stimulation to the brain after FPI has been observed to elicit a metabolic response that may act as a secondary injury by increasing cortical degeneration.[62] Metabolic and ionic disturbances also affect function of the N-methyl-D-aspartate receptor (NMDAR), which is a key molecular player in neuronal activation and allows for long-term potentiation (LTP), a cellular correlate of learning. As a glutamate receptor, the NMDAR plays a major role in neuronal excitability. The response to injury, such as the period of metabolic depression, differs between adult and developing animals.[5,63,64]

Changes in brain activation can also have an effect on the regulation of the hypothalamic pituitary adrenal (HPA) axis. Efficient HPA regulation is necessary for neuronal vitality and function, thus its dysregulation can have profound effects on synaptic plasticity as well as cognitive and affective well-being. Glucocorticoid release is regulated by the hypothalamus, a region receiving multiple suprahypothalamic inputs with notable projections from the limbic system. Alterations in function and connectivity are likely to exert a substantial influence on HPA regulation. Glucocorticoid receptors are widespread throughout the brain and are predominantly expressed within the hippocampus.[65,66] Excitatory changes within the hippocampus thus have an effect on glucorticoid negative feedback. Recent findings from adult rodent studies indicate that there is a hyperresponsiveness to stress after a mild FPI. This hyperresponsiveness was observed during the first postinjury weeks.[67] These increases indicate hypothalamic disruptions in neuronal circuitry. A heightening of the stress response may be particularly concerning in the developing brain. Neonatal or pubertal stress has a pronounced effect on adult behavior and brain plasticity.[68–70] Along these lines, corticotropin-releasing hormone mRNA has been shown to increase after TBI.[71,72] In addition to the heightened stress response, animal studies, using different injury models, have indicated other TBI-induced changes in HPA regulation.[73,74]

Human Studies

As shown in animal models of injury, neurochemical and metabolic disruptions are also observed in humans. Metabolic disruptions after experimental TBI extend over a period of days and normalize after approximately 10 days,[11,12] whereas changes after moderate to severe human TBI may last weeks or even months.[75] In addition, the consequences stemming from a TBI include white matter damage and changes in activation patterns. These alterations are likely to contribute to the long-term cognitive impairments that are observed after TBI. These impairments range from acute memory problems to difficulty with higher executive functions such as strategy switching and planning. A functional magnetic resonance imaging (MRI) study of individuals with mild or moderate brain injury found neural activity alterations a year after injury. In particular, disruptions in catecholaminergic circuitry, which is associated with working memory functions, were observed.[76] Alterations in activation after mild brain injury are also associated with axonal damage, but this is generally not apparent with computed tomography.[77] Subtle white matter abnormalities are observed in patients with persistent postconcussive symptoms after suffering from a mild TBI using diffusion tensor imaging (DTI) (see later discussion).[78]

As indicated earlier, changes in activation patterns are likely to have an effect on glucocorticoid regulation. Acute activation of the HPA axis occurs initially after brain injury as a protective response that modulates the immune/inflammatory response and increases metabolic substrate availability.[79] Clinical studies have shown increases in cortisol acutely after brain trauma and these increases are correlated with the duration of coma and recovery after head trauma.[62,80] As for the subacute period, studies suggest that plasma cortisol levels are dependent on the injury severity. Cortisol tends to increase after mild to moderate brain injury in the early post-injury period, whereas it is depressed after a severe injury.[81,82] Although structural pituitary damage may be dependent on the severity of the injury,[83] pituitary abnormalities have been reported in mild to moderate injuries. MRI studies indicate that 37% of adult patients with mild TBI, with a Glasgow coma score ranging from 13 to 15, had structural pituitary abnormalities.[84] A higher rate of pituitary abnormalities was found in a pediatric study looking at functional measures. Basal cortisol levels were significantly reduced in this population.[85] It still remains to be answered if there is an age-dependent vulnerability of the HPA axis.

ALTERED PLASTICITY AND DEVELOPMENT
Experimental

Brain injury leads to alterations in molecular substrates of synaptic plasticity. Of particular interest are the effects on proteins such as BDNF and the NMDAR, which are strongly linked with synaptic strengthening and play a significant role in experience-dependent plasticity.[86,87] Because the young brain is undergoing developmental changes, injury-induced alterations of molecular markers of plasticity may not only affect injury outcome, as it has been shown in adults, but also deviate developmental processes from their normal trajectory.

It is during the developmental period that the brain is more susceptible to environmental influences. This finding has been shown in enriched environment (EE) studies. These studies indicate that structural changes are more likely to occur in a developing rat as a response to environmental stimulation when compared with an adult rat.[88–90] However, when a developing rat is exposed to an EE after a FPI, the beneficial effects that indicate neuroplasticity, such as cortical thickening, expanded dendritic arborization, and cognitive enhancement, are not observed.[91,92] The cognitive benefit that is usually found after EE exposure is found only if the period of enrichment is delayed after the injury.[93] This failure to enrich after developmental TBI is observed despite no significant cell death.[94] This finding shows that mechanisms driving neuroplasticity are affected after TBI and may lead to the failure to appropriately respond to environmental stimulation. In accordance with this idea, changes in NMDAR composition have been observed after an FPI in young rats.[95] In addition, alterations in molecules that facilitate synaptic plasticity, such as BDNF, are likely contributors to the post-TBI failure of EE.

Adult TBI studies have shown that expression of BDNF is acutely altered in different models of TBI.[96–99] BDNF mRNA is dynamically regulated during postnatal development in various central nervous system structures and its levels are high and unstable compared with the mature brain.[100–102] Therefore, it is plausible that the effects of TBI on BDNF are age dependent. Levels of BDNF were observed to be increased after an FPI in developing rats when compared with adult FPI.[103,104] These increases in BDNF were most pronounced in areas remote from the injury site and may indicate synaptic remodeling. Reorganization after brain injury has been proposed as a mechanism to facilitate recovery[105–107] and has been observed in animals after brain injury.[58,92,108–111]

A substantial increase in neuronal connectivity occurs during the postnatal period, as a response to functional and environmental demands. During this period, the organization of fiber projections takes place through regionally selective outgrowth or selective elimination of projections.[112,113] These ongoing maturational processes emphasize the significance of TBI studies in this age range. These studies suggest that after TBI, future developmental plasticity may be compromised, in that neuroplasticity shifts from responding to experience-dependent adaptation to that of restoration/compensation to a preinjury status.

Human Studies

Data obtained from human TBI studies indicates that the capacity of the brain to compensate for injury is largely dependent on the state of cerebral maturation. For example, children younger than 4 years have a worse outcome compared with older children.[114,115] Paradoxically, although children may be more behaviorally resilient to injury, cognitive deficits may not be noticeable until the child is exposed to a more demanding environment. Thus, deficits in attention, memory, and verbal abilities may become apparent only later in development; these impairments after pediatric TBI may also manifest as an increased likelihood of needing special education programs.[116–118]

The brain is rapidly developing during the first years. Events refining neural connectivity are actively taking place through processes such as myelination, dendritic changes, and synaptogenesis.[119] As suggested by the animal literature, TBI in young children jeopardizes ongoing developmental processes.[120,121] Studies by Anderson and colleagues[115,122] indicate that executive functions, such as information processing and the ability to suppress impulsive behaviors, are particularly affected in those children who suffered a TBI before the age of 3 years. Deficits in executive functions were observed regardless of injury location[123]; thus suggesting that the alteration of neural networks caused by injury had an effect on skills that are acquired at a future developmental period. With the exception of attentional control, it was the skills that were in the process of being acquired at the time of injury that were more likely to show impairments. A recent study of young adults who had suffered from a TBI during childhood indicates that these impairments may be long lasting, particularly after a severe TBI. In these individuals quality of life and employment opportunities were reduced.[124]

TIMING OF RETURN TO ACTIVITY

As discussed earlier, there is substantial evidence that neural activation and plasticity are altered after developmental TBI. It is also known that physiologic neural activation can promote recovery, whereas excessive activation may exacerbate cellular damage. These neurobiological principles, then, underlie the clinically relevant determination of the optimal timing for return to activity after TBI/concussion.

Experimental

Ideally exercise should facilitate the capacity of the brain to compensate for insults, thus resulting in a better outcome. Numerous studies have shown that exercise, particularly of a voluntary nature, increases markers of neuroplasticity and promotes neurogenesis.[60,125–130] However, this situation may not always be the case if particular considerations are not taken into account when implementing exercise in the postconcussive setting.

Animal studies have shown that the beneficial effects of exercise are found only if exercise is delayed after TBI. In these studies, rodents underwent a mild FPI and were allowed to exercise for a week, starting on the day of the injury. Not only did these rats fail to show an increase in BDNF and other target proteins but also presented cognitive deterioration when compared with their sedentary counterparts.[61] Moreover, experimental findings suggested that premature exercise disrupts restorative processes. Proteins associated with plasticity that were increased as a result of TBI, in areas remote from the site of injury, were reduced when rats were acutely exercised.[103] Compensatory or restorative responses may be observed in areas of the brain that have endured a lesser amount of harm.[105–107,131–134]

In contrast to acute postinjury exercise, when exercise was delayed after an FPI, increases in BDNF were observed. This exercise-induced increase in BDNF was associated with enhanced hippocampal-dependent learning and memory.[135] A cognitive benefit is typically observed as a result of voluntary exercise.[136] In addition to BDNF, exercise increases other proteins that enhance neural function and cognitive performance. Some of these proteins have been found to increase with exercise after experimental brain injury. For example calcium-calmodulin-dependent protein kinase II (CaMKII) and cyclic adenosine monophosphate response-element-binding protein (CREB) are increased when postinjury exercise is delayed. Both of these have substances been shown to facilitate LTP, a key cellular mechanism underlying synaptic plasticity and learning. In addition, animal studies suggest that this time window is dependent on the particular characteristics of the injury; for example, the necessary delay for exercise to be effective after an FPI is severity dependent.[137]

Although it is still unknown why the injured brain does not respond to acute postinjury exercise it is plausible that untimely exercise may divert cerebral metabolism from needed functions such as energy restoration and production of synaptic plasticity molecules, by introducing an increase in metabolic demand at a time when the brain is energetically compromised. TBI results in mitochondrial dysfunction and decreases in blood flow that compromise neuronal functioning and signaling. These disruptions in cellular function along with injury-induced changes in activation are likely to interfere with the effects of exercise.

In addition, as indicated earlier, TBI disrupts the regulation of stress hormones, and may heighten the stress response for the first postinjury weeks. Glucocorticoids, which are known to suppress levels of BDNF and other key proteins,[106,138–142] may have increased levels after injury and contribute to the undesired effects of early postinjury exercise. In addition, a hyperresponse to stress is likely to magnify regular metabolic effects of exercise. Exercise by itself places an energetic demand and moderately increases levels of corticosteroids.[143,144] Some forms of exercise elicit a stronger stress response. Different forms of exercise involve distinct motivational and fatigue characteristics. Thus certain exercise regimens with stronger stress responses may be particularly counterproductive during the early postinjury period.

Human Studies

As in animal studies, neuroprotective qualities have been associated with exercise in humans. There is a wealth of studies indicating the beneficial effects of exercise on cognitive function and mental health.[145–149] In children, exercise is associated with improved academic performance and executive functioning.[150-153] Exercise has also been found to decrease headaches,[154,155] which are one of the main symptoms reported after mild TBI in both children and adults.

The effects of exercise have also been explored in the TBI population. A retrospective study that relied on self-reports found that postinjury exercise decreased negative mood states in adults.[156] Affective disorders are prevalent in the population with TBI.[157,158] Another study found that the practice of aquatic activities, at least 12 months after TBI, decreased the incidence of negative moods.[159] Although most of the exercise studies assessing postconcussive effects have been in adults, it is also likely that the benefits of exercise are present in a younger population. A review of different trials with patients after TBI ranging in age from 3 to 20 years found a short-term improvement in self-esteem.[160] Other studies have found that exercise lessens postconcussive symptoms, such as headaches, dizziness, and fatigue.[161] Gagnon and colleagues' study used gradual and controlled exercise rehabilitation in a pediatric population with TBI who presented symptoms 4 to 18 weeks after TBI.

Exercise studies in the population with TBI have included a wide range of postinjury periods, but few offered observations acutely after injury. Among these, a retrospective cohort study by Majerske and colleagues[162] found that high levels of cognitive and physical activity during the early postinjury period had a negative effect on cognitive function and were associated with worsened concussive symptoms and performance on cognitive testing. The occurrence of negative mood states and cognitive impairments may be associated with neuroendocrine alterations that are found in the early post-TBI weeks, such as increased plasma cortisol levels.[82]

These findings indicate that premature neural activation alone, without a repeated injury, can have a deleterious effect. Thus it is not only the risk of a repeated concussion that is of concern when addressing the return to play but also the potential deleterious effect of excessive, early neural activity. When a second concussion occurs the brain is more susceptible to damage as a result of ongoing conditions from the first injury.[39,163,164] Because of these concerns, consensus guidelines for the reinstatement of physical activities after TBI[165-167] recommend avoiding activities such as physical and cognitive exertion until postconcussive symptoms have resolved. Determining the optimal time for return to activity can be challenging in the sports or military setting. Having fixed waiting guidelines may be too conservative or not sufficient, because injury characteristics and recovery vary greatly between patients. However, symptom resolution may not always be self-reported accurately, nor may it reflect full cerebral or neurocognitive recovery.[23,168,169] The timeline for effective exercise therapy as well as return to physical activities is dependent on the characteristics of the injury as well as previous injury history and thus should be tailored on an individual basis. Because of these concerns it is important to understand the physiologic and neurobehavioral correlates that underlie the injury. The literature regarding therapeutic exercise is largely based on anecdotal data and randomized studies on patients with TBI are sparse, indicating a pressing need for further rigorous investigations.

AXONAL INJURY
Experimental

It is well known that biomechanical forces applied to neural tissue result in dysfunction and damage to axons.[170-172] Changes in axonal integrity and function have been described in experimental models of mild TBI,[39] including a recently described model of repeat concussive injury in the juvenile rat.[26] In this juvenile model, the degree of axonal damage and glial reactivity was amplified when 2 closed head injuries were experienced 1 day apart. Behaviorally, a single mild TBI caused a decrement in working memory that was worsened by the combined injury.

Another consideration when investigating axonal damage during development is that myelination is ongoing in many brain regions throughout cerebral maturation. There is evidence that unmyelinated fibers may be more vulnerable to TBI, as shown by Reeves and colleagues.[173] In that study, midline FPI resulted in a loss of compound action potentials through the corpus callosum, and, although recovery of the myelinated fibers occurred over time, persistent deficits in the unmyelinated peaks were seen. These data suggest that unmyelinated axons, and thus immature axons, could be more vulnerable to biomechanical injuries.

Imaging of animal TBI models provides insight into axonal injury. For example, DTI, an advanced MRI technique that measures directional diffusion as a marker of white matter fiber integrity, has been studied after experimental controlled cortical impact injury. Changes in DTI signal have been correlated with histopathologic findings.[174,175]

Human Studies

In the adult brain, there is substantial pathologic evidence for axonal injury after severe TBI,[176,177] but only a few such reports of axonal damage after milder, concussive injury, which were in older persons.[178,179] Advances in noninvasive neuroimaging, particularly DTI, have provided new insight into white matter damage or dysfunction occurring after TBI, including in the pediatric and young adult population.[180–183] Fractional anisotropy (FA) is a measure of the directionality of water diffusion, with a value of 1 being the highest, and a value of 0 indicating diffusion equally in all directions (essentially no directionality).

In children with moderate to severe TBI compared with orthopedic controls, DTI showed abnormalities in frontal white matter 3 months after injury. These abnormalities, such as decreased FA, were predictive of long-term global outcomes.[181] Similar reductions of FA were reported in the corpus callosa (CC) of adolescents after moderate to severe TBI, which was also correlated with reduced CC NAA on MRS.[184]

Studies of DTI after mild TBI/sports concussions have been limited to older adolescents and adults (for review of DTI methods in general, see Ref.[185]) An early pediatric DTI study compared control subjects with those with mild and moderate TBI (average age 15.1 ± 2.3 years, postinjury time 8.2 ± 2.2 months). This study showed lower FA values in children with moderate TBI and neurocognitive impairments in the combined mild to moderate TBI group.[180] Specifically in the supracallosal region, both mild and moderate groups separately showed significantly reduced FA compared with controls. Wilde and colleagues[182] measured DTI in adolescents within the first week after concussion and showed increased FA in corpus callosum, which correlated strongly with the clinical scores on the Rivermead post concussion symptom questionnaire (RPCSQ). This increased FA was postulated to indicate early axonal swelling, which favors diffusion along the direction of the callosal fibers. Using multimodal imaging combining DTI and magnetoencephalography (MEG), a group of young military and civilian adults with postconcussion symptoms and normal conventional neuroimaging were studied. This study showed areas of decreased FA in subcortical white matter underlying areas of focal slowing on MEG[183] and supported the usefulness of this combined imaging methodology to distinguish between patients with mild TBI and controls.

It is likely that both DTI and MRS of white matter fibers will yield greater insight into postconcussion axonal pathobiology. Such noninvasive scans may be readily conducted in humans, and translational work investigating MRI and histopathology in experimental animal models will greatly aid in the elucidating mechanisms underlying abnormal white matter signals on advanced MRI sequences. Further critical work is also required in establishing clinical correlates of these white matter abnormalities, determining the longitudinal time course of axonal injury and distinguishing differences in traumatic axonal injury between the pediatric and adult brain.

CHRONIC TRAUMATIC ENCEPHALOPATHY AND LATE RISK OF DEMENTIA

Chronic traumatic encephalopathy is a progressive neurodegenerative disease found in some individuals subjected to repetitive mild TBI. Neuropathologically, it can be described as a tauopathy of the brain manifesting as neurofibrillary tangles throughout most of the brain with a relative paucity of β-amyloid deposition.[186]

Experimental

Single and recurrent mild TBI and the effect on amyloid proteins associated with dementia have been extensively studied in animal models. Most research has focused on Aβ-amyloid accumulation and its correlation with cognitive impairment. Increased levels of amyloid precursor protein (APP) have been found in animals undergoing recurrent TBI,[187] as well as increased levels of β-secretase[188] and γ-secretase enzymes,[189] which are both known to convert APP into neurotoxic Aβ peptides. Likely related to these findings, Aβ1-40 and Aβ1-42 levels have also been found to be significantly increased in the hippocampal neurons of PDAPP transgenic mice overexpressing mutant human APP who are subjected to cortical impact brain injury compared with noninjured transgenic mice. The injured hippocampi showed substantial exacerbation of neuronal death, which suggests that there is a mechanistic link between brain trauma, Aβ levels, and neuronal cell death.[190] With repetitive mild TBI in Tg APP695swe (Tg2576) transgenic mice that overexpress mutant APP, accelerated deposition of Aβ plaques and earlier onset of cognitive impairment are also seen.[191] Research with nontransgenic mice has shown that after controlled cortical impact, accumulation of mouse Aβx-40 peptide was noted after 1 day, with increasing levels of almost 120% seen by 3 days, and normalization of levels by 7 days.[192] Other evidence supporting the involvement of Aβ plaque formation in long-term outcomes comes from research performed by exposing pigs to inertial brain injury, which was found to cause long-term (up to 6 months after injury) accumulation of APP, β-site APP cleaving enzyme, presenilin 1, and activated caspase in the axons of injured neurons. The accumulation of these factors is believed to be caused by impaired axonal transport because of trauma, and it may lead to APP proteolysis and Aβ formation within the axonal membrane compartment.[193] Postconcussive Aβ plaque formation may help to explain the increased risk of Alzheimer disease after mild TBI through acceleration of the postulated amyloid cascade.[194]

Gross Pathology

Individuals with a history of multiple episodes of mild TBI may have 1 or several stigmata associated with repetitive concussion. Often seen are such findings as an anterior septum pellucidum cavum, as well as posterior fenestrations in the ventricular system.[195] Individuals with septum pellucidum cavum may also develop recurrent obstructive hydrocephalus as a result of abnormalities in cerebrospinal fluid (CSF) flow, requiring ventricular fenestration or ventriculoperitoneal shunt placement.[196] Other gross pathologic conditions includes atrophy of the frontotemporal cortex, medial temporal lobe, hypothalamic floor, and mammillary bodies, as well as enlargement of the third and lateral ventricles, hippocampal sclerosis, and pallor of the substantia nigra. A reduction in total brain volume may be seen, with atrophy noted in the cerebrum, diencephalon, basal ganglia, and brainstem.[186]

Microscopic Pathology

Several different microscopic findings are seen with repetitive chronic mild TBI, including tau-positive neurofibrillary tangles, astrocytic/glial tangles, and neurites of spindle and threadlike shapes. Deposition of β-amyloid occurs in less than half of cases, according to 1 retrospective study.[186] In addition, recent attention has been drawn to the potential involvement of transactive response (TAR) DNA binding protein-43kDa (TDP-43) in the pathophysiology of chronic traumatic encephalopathy.[197] Diffuse cerebral white matter degeneration has long been known to occur with severe dementia after head injury.[198] Multifocal axonal injury with damage in the corpus callosum and the fornices has been rarely described after single mild TBI in patients who died shortly after injury as a result of nonneurologic complications.[178] Gross fornix degeneration has also been noted in similar patients.[199]

Tau-based Protein Deposits

Historically, neurofibrillary tangles, mostly comprised of tau protein, have been regularly seen in the brains of patients with a history of multiple mild traumatic brain injuries. The exact mechanism that leads to their accumulation is not known. As mentioned earlier, shearing forces acting on neuronal axons lead to increased cell membrane permeability, ionic disequilibrium, and often trigger intracellular apoptotic enzymes, which may initiate and later aggravate formation of neurofibrillary tangles via tau truncation, phosphorylation, and misfolding.[170,171,200] Also contributing to their production and accumulation is cytoskeletal element breakdown, notably microtubules and microfilaments.[201]

Neurofibrillary tangles are seen predominantly in the superficial cortex (layer II and the upper portion of layer III), mostly in frontotemporal and insular distributions.[202] They are generally found in patches, notably in the deeper portions of the sulci as well as subpial, periventricular, and perivascular areas.[186,203] They are often seen with neuritic threads, seen in the subcortical nuclei/basal ganglia, hippocampus, brainstem nuclei, and cerebral cortices,[204] with notable cortical involvement of the frontal and temporal lobes, as well as the insula.[186] According to McKee and colleagues,[186] both neurofibrillary and glial tangles were found in the medial temporal lobe, diencephalon, brain stem, and basal ganglia, as well as subcortical white matter of subjects with chronic traumatic encephalopathy. The perivascular distribution of neurofibrillary tangles suggests that mechanical disruption of the cerebral microvasculature may play a role in their deposition. These distributions remarkably contrast those of Alzheimer disease, which are generally seen in a more uniform cortical distribution, mostly in cortical layers III and V, without perivascular predominance.

Extension of the tau-based neurofibrillary tangles from the isolated perivascular spaces to broader, patchy distributions is not completely understood; however, some evidence suggests misfolded tau proteins are able to propagate out of 1 cell and into another, similar to prions. This phenomenon has been observed in vitro and is described as extracellular tau aggregate being taken up by cultured cells and internalized, leading to fibrillization of new tau proteins intracellularly via displacement of tubulin and colocalization with dextran.[205]

β-Amyloid (Aβ) Deposits

Neuritic β-amyloid plaques are seen in slightly less than half of all cases of chronic traumatic encephalopathy. Their distribution differs markedly from those found in

Alzheimer disease, because patients with multiple concussions show diffuse plaques with less density than the abundant plaques seen in Alzheimer disease.[186] Although the pathogenesis of β-amyloid deposits is not entirely clear, APP has been found to accumulate in the axonal bulbs of injured neurons after diffuse axonal injury, as seen in mild TBI, most commonly in subcortical and deep white matter.[206] APP is then likely cleaved to form β-amyloid. There is conflicting evidence regarding the exact role played by β-amyloid in pathogenesis versus neuroprotection in injured neurons.[206,207]

TAR TDP-43

A recent study reported neuropathologic evidence for the theoretic epidemiologic linkage between head injury and amyotrophic lateral sclerosis. A small number of cases with chronic traumatic encephalopathy and severe motor neuron disease were found to have TDP-43 deposits in the brain as well as in the anterior horns of the spinal cord.[197] The conclusions drawn from these results, most notably a link between repetitive mild TBI and amyotrophic lateral sclerosis, remain controversial.[208,209]

CSF Markers of Repetitive Head Trauma

Short-term biochemical aberrations in the face of head trauma have been investigated. CSF markers of repetitive head trauma (neurofilament light protein, total tau, glial fibrillary acidic protein [GFAP], phosphorylated tau, and β-amyloid protein 1-40 and 1-42) have been studied in amateur boxers at 7 to 10 days and 3 months after fight and compared with healthy, nonathletic controls. Neurofilament light protein, total tau, and fibrillary acidic protein were found to be increased shortly after fights compared with 3 months later in boxers, with the increase dramatically higher among those receiving more punches or more high-impact hits to the head. Compared with controls, the boxers had significantly higher levels of neurofilament light protein and GFAP 7 to 10 days after a fight. Neurofilament light protein was the only CSF marker found to be significantly increased 3 months after a fight in boxers compared with controls.[210]

Other CSF biomarkers have been identified and found to be altered long-term in those with repetitive head trauma. Zetterberg and colleagues[211] compared CSF levels of S-100B, BDNF, heart-type fatty acid binding protein, GFAP, and neuron-specific enolase using biochip array in amateur boxers after 2 months of boxing abstention compared with healthy controls with no history of head trauma. These investigators found that only neuron-specific enolase was significantly increased, whereas the remainder of the CSF markers tested showed no differences between the boxers and controls. Finding no significant differences in CSF tau concentrations between resting boxers and controls supports CSF tau as a biomarker of acute concussive injury and not chronic repetitive mild brain trauma. Alterations in neurofilament light protein were not mentioned in the 2009 study.

Genetic Susceptibility to Chronic Traumatic Encephalopathy

In addition to the neuropathologic similarities between chronic traumatic encephalopathy and Alzheimer disease mentioned earlier, the genetics predisposing to both disorders also seem to have significant overlap. It is well known that apolipoprotein E is a susceptibility gene for late-onset familial and sporadic Alzheimer disease, and that possessing the ε4 genotype leads to dose-dependent hastening of the onset of Alzheimer disease.[212–214] The development of chronic traumatic encephalopathy has also been linked to the ε4 genotype.[215] Having the same apolipoprotein E ε4 genotype also predisposes the individual to incurring significantly more severe chronic traumatic encephalopathy compared with those without the ε4 genotype, given the same degree of chronic TBI.[216] It is unknown whether possessing the apolipoprotein E ε2 genotype is protective in chronic traumatic encephalopathy, as it seems to be in Alzheimer disease.[217] The implications of these findings support the theory that chronic traumatic encephalopathy, as well as Alzheimer disease, share a complex combination of both environmental and genetic risk factors. Future consideration should be given to the possibility of genetic counseling for professional athletes likely to encounter repeated head trauma and their likelihood of developing an encephalopathic state.

SUMMARY

Our understanding of the phenomenon of concussion has been shaped significantly by experimental work in animal models, as well as extrapolation of physiologic measurements from humans with more severe TBI. This review covers 3 main postconcussive periods: (1) the acute neurometabolic cascade, (2) the subacute phase of altered neural activation and axonal disconnection, and (3) the chronic accumulation of insults that may lead to permanent impairments. The acute neurometabolic cascade involves indiscriminate neurotransmitter release, ionic disequilibrium, metabolic crisis (with energy depletion and oxidative stress), and cytoskeletal damage. These pathophysiologic alterations also occur after mild TBI and create a state of vulnerability to repeated injury. In animals, these acute neurometabolic perturbations may take 7 to 10 days to recover fully. In humans, abnormal metabolic patterns seen on MRS after mild TBI may require up to 4 weeks to recover. Beyond the acute changes, concussive brain injury is followed by a period of impaired neuroplasticity and axonal disconnection. Both of these phenomena may have significant implications for recovery when they occur or recur in the immature brain, because they may result in a slowed developmental trajectory, with persistent or emergent neurocognitive deficits that only fully manifest over time. After mild TBI, experimental evidence indicates that not only is the concussed brain less responsive to physiologic neural activation, but it may also be more vulnerable to premature forced activation that can act as a secondary stressor to exacerbate dysfunction and neural damage. These findings correlate loosely with clinical data suggesting that repeated concussions or excessive levels of postinjury activity lead to longer duration and greater severity of postconcussive symptoms. Together, these preclinical and clinical data form the basis for consensus recommendations of delayed return to activity and return to play. There is growing evidence for chronic, cumulative neurobiological impairment, centered on abnormal protein deposition, delayed cell death and axotomy, and resultant cognitive and behavioral decline.

Knowledge of these cellular mechanisms is important for understanding the distinctions of concussions as they occur in children and adolescents. First, the young brain may be biologically more vulnerable to repeat mild TBI, through impairments in neural activation/plasticity and increased sensitivity of developing axons to biomechanical forces. Second, the population of young children exposed to contact sports is relatively unselected genetically, and thus, genetic risk factors for worsened acute symptoms have not yet been weaned out, as they may be in more elite collegiate or professional adult athletic populations. Third, the risk of cumulative damage may be mathematically linked to duration of exposure, which is logically greater when exposure to concussions begins at a younger age. Last, it is important to understand that many cognitive functions are not yet fully developed in pediatric populations, and thus, cognitive assessment tools designed for adults may have significant limitations when applied to young athletes. Although mild TBI/concussion and repeated traumatic injuries associated with sports occur frequently in these younger populations, there is still a dearth of clinical data in grade school and junior high school age children. Considering all these factors related to youth concussion, it is most reasonable to approach the clinical management and return to play for these individuals more conservatively than adults, and to call for more translational work targeting both the short-term and long-term effects of repeated mild TBI in the developing brain.

ACKNOWLEDGMENTS

NS27544, NS057420, NS06190, the Child Neurology Foundation/Winokur Family Foundation, the Today's and Tomorrow's Children Fund, and UCLA Brain Injury Research Center.

REFERENCES

1. Langlois JA, Rutland-Brown W, Thomas KE. The incidence of traumatic brain injury among children in the United States: differences by race. J Head Trauma Rehabil 2005;20(3):229–38.
2. Farkas O, Lifshitz J, Povlishock JT. Mechanoporation induced by diffuse traumatic brain injury: an irreversible or reversible response to injury? J Neurosci 2006;26(12):3130–40.
3. Katayama Y, Becker DP, Tamura T, et al. Massive increases in extracellular potassium and the indiscriminate release of glutamate following concussive brain injury. J Neurosurg 1990;73(6):889–900.
4. Osteen CL, Giza CC, Hovda DA. Injury-induced alterations in N-methyl-D-aspartate receptor subunit composition contribute to prolonged 45calcium accumulation following lateral fluid percussion. Neuroscience 2004;128(2):305–22.
5. Osteen CL, Moore AH, Prins ML, et al. Age-dependency of 45calcium accumulation following lateral fluid percussion: acute and delayed patterns. J Neurotrauma 2001;18(2):141–62.
6. Fineman I, Hovda DA, Smith M, et al. Concussive brain injury is associated with a prolonged accumulation of calcium: a 45Ca autoradiographic study. Brain Res 1993;624(1-2):94–102.
7. Raghupathi R. Cell death mechanisms following traumatic brain injury. Brain Pathol 2004;14(2):215–22.
8. Sullivan PG, Rabchevsky AG, Waldmeier PC, et al. Mitochondrial permeability transition in CNS trauma: cause or effect of neuronal cell death? J Neurosci Res 2005;79(1-2):231–9.
9. Reinert M, Hoelper B, Doppenberg E, et al. Substrate delivery and ionic balance disturbance after severe human head injury. Acta Neurochir Suppl 2000;76: 439–44.
10. Yuen TJ, Browne KD, Iwata A, et al. Sodium channelopathy induced by mild axonal trauma worsens outcome after a repeat injury. J Neurosci Res 2009; 87(16):3620–5.
11. Yoshino A, Hovda DA, Kawamata T, et al. Dynamic changes in local cerebral glucose utilization following cerebral concussion in rats: evidence of a hyper- and subsequent hypometabolic state. Brain Res 1991;561(1):106–19.
12. Kawamata T, Katayama Y, Hovda DA, et al. Lactate accumulation following concussive brain injury: the role of ionic fluxes induced by excitatory amino acids. Brain Res 1995;674(2):196–204.

13. Kalimo H, Rehncrona S, Soderfeldt B. The role of lactic acidosis in the ischemic nerve cell injury. Acta Neuropathol Suppl 1981;7:20–2.
14. Glenn TC, Kelly DF, Boscardin WJ, et al. Energy dysfunction as a predictor of outcome after moderate or severe head injury: indices of oxygen, glucose, and lactate metabolism. J Cereb Blood Flow Metab 2003;23(10):1239–50.
15. Martin NA, Patwardhan RV, Alexander MJ, et al. Characterization of cerebral hemodynamic phases following severe head trauma: hypoperfusion, hyperemia, and vasospasm. J Neurosurg 1997;87(1):9–19.
16. Golding EM, Steenberg ML, Contant CF Jr, et al. Cerebrovascular reactivity to CO(2) and hypotension after mild cortical impact injury. Am J Physiol 1999; 277(4 Pt 2):H1457–66.
17. Grindel SH. Epidemiology and pathophysiology of minor traumatic brain injury. Curr Sports Med Rep 2003;2(1):18–23.
18. Chan KH, Miller JD, Dearden NM. Intracranial blood flow velocity after head injury: relationship to severity of injury, time, neurological status and outcome. J Neurol Neurosurg Psychiatry 1992;55(9):787–91.
19. Mandera M, Larysz D, Wojtacha M. Changes in cerebral hemodynamics assessed by transcranial Doppler ultrasonography in children after head injury. Childs Nerv Syst 2002;18(3-4):124–8.
20. Becelewski J, Pierzchala K. [Cerebrovascular reactivity in patients with mild head injury]. Neurol Neurochir Pol 2003;37(2):339–50 [in Polish].
21. Vavilala MS, Lee LA, Boddu K, et al. Cerebral autoregulation in pediatric traumatic brain injury. Pediatr Crit Care Med 2004;5(3):257–63.
22. Chaiwat O, Sharma D, Udomphorn Y, et al. Cerebral hemodynamic predictors of poor 6-month Glasgow Outcome Score in severe pediatric traumatic brain injury. J Neurotrauma 2009;26(5):657–63.
23. Vagnozzi R, Signoretti S, Tavazzi B, et al. Temporal window of metabolic brain vulnerability to concussion: a pilot 1H-magnetic resonance spectroscopic study in concussed athletes–part III. Neurosurgery 2008;62(6):1286–95 [discussion: 1295–6].
24. Tavazzi B, Vagnozzi R, Signoretti S, et al. Temporal window of metabolic brain vulnerability to concussions: oxidative and nitrosative stresses–part II. Neurosurgery 2007;61(2):390–5.
25. Vagnozzi R, Tavazzi B, Signoretti S, et al. Temporal window of metabolic brain vulnerability to concussions: mitochondrial-related impairment–part I. Neurosurgery 2007;61(2):379–88.
26. Prins ML, Hales A, Reger M, et al. Repeat traumatic brain injury in the juvenile rat is associated with increased axonal injury and cognitive impairments. Dev Neurosci 2010;32(5-6):510–8.
27. Putukian M. Repeat mild traumatic brain injury: how to adjust return to play guidelines. Curr Sports Med Rep 2006;5(1):15–22.
28. Kissick J, Johnston KM. Return to play after concussion: principles and practice. Clin J Sport Med 2005;15(6):426–31.
29. Guskiewicz KM, McCrea M, Marshall SW, et al. Cumulative effects associated with recurrent concussion in collegiate football players: the NCAA Concussion Study. JAMA 2003;290(19):2549–55.
30. Saunders RL, Harbaugh RE. The second impact in catastrophic contact-sports head trauma. JAMA 1984;252(4):538–9.
31. Cantu RC. Second-impact syndrome. Clin Sports Med 1998;17(1):37–44.
32. McCrory PR, Berkovic SF. Second impact syndrome. Neurology 1998;50(3): 677–83.

33. Wetjen NM, Pichelmann MA, Atkinson JL. Second impact syndrome: concussion and second injury brain complications. J Am Coll Surg 2010;211(4):553–7.
34. Clifton GL, Ziegler MG, Grossman RG. Circulating catecholamines and sympathetic activity after head injury. Neurosurgery 1981;8(1):10–4.
35. Lam JM, Hsiang JN, Poon WS. Monitoring of autoregulation using laser Doppler flowmetry in patients with head injury. J Neurosurg 1997;86(3):438–45.
36. McCrory P. Does second impact syndrome exist? Clin J Sport Med 2001;11(3): 144–9.
37. Cantu RC, Gean AD. Second-impact syndrome and a small subdural hematoma: an uncommon catastrophic result of repetitive head injury with a characteristic imaging appearance. J Neurotrauma 2010;27(9):1557–64.
38. Kors EE, Terwindt GM, Vermeulen FL, et al. Delayed cerebral edema and fatal coma after minor head trauma: role of the CACNA1A calcium channel subunit gene and relationship with familial hemiplegic migraine. Ann Neurol 2001; 49(6):753–60.
39. Longhi L, Saatman KE, Fujimoto S, et al. Temporal window of vulnerability to repetitive experimental concussive brain injury. Neurosurgery 2005;56(2): 364–74 [discussion: 364–74].
40. Doberstein CE, Hovda DA, Becker DP. Clinical considerations in the reduction of secondary brain injury. Ann Emerg Med 1993;22(6):993–7.
41. Vagnozzi R, Signoretti S, Tavazzi B, et al. Hypothesis of the postconcussive vulnerable brain: experimental evidence of its metabolic occurrence. Neurosurgery 2005;57(1):164–71.
42. Creeley CE, Wozniak DF, Bayly PV, et al. Multiple episodes of mild traumatic brain injury result in impaired cognitive performance in mice. Acad Emerg Med 2004;11(8):809–19.
43. Garnett MR, Blamire AM, Corkill RG, et al. Early proton magnetic resonance spectroscopy in normal-appearing brain correlates with outcome in patients following traumatic brain injury. Brain 2000;123(Pt 10):2046–54.
44. Garnett MR, Blamire AM, Rajagopalan B, et al. Evidence for cellular damage in normal-appearing white matter correlates with injury severity in patients following traumatic brain injury: a magnetic resonance spectroscopy study. Brain 2000;123(Pt 7):1403–9.
45. Tran LD, Lifshitz J, Witgen BM, et al. Response of the contralateral hippocampus to lateral fluid percussion brain injury. J Neurotrauma 2006;23(9):1330–42.
46. Avramescu S, Timofeev I. Synaptic strength modulation after cortical trauma: a role in epileptogenesis. J Neurosci 2008;28(27):6760–72.
47. Salin P, Tseng GF, Hoffman S, et al. Axonal sprouting in layer V pyramidal neurons of chronically injured cerebral cortex. J Neurosci 1995;15(12):8234–45.
48. Topolnik L, Steriade M, Timofeev I. Hyperexcitability of intact neurons underlies acute development of trauma-related electrographic seizures in cats in vivo. Eur J Neurosci 2003;18(3):486–96.
49. Dinner DS. Posttraumatic epilepsy. In: Wyllie E, editor. The treatment of epilepsy: principles. Philadelphia: Lea & Febiger; 1993. p. 654–8.
50. Bergsneider M, Hovda DA, Lee SM, et al. Dissociation of cerebral glucose metabolism and level of consciousness during the period of metabolic depression following human traumatic brain injury. J Neurotrauma 2000;17(5): 389–401.
51. Ginsberg MD, Zhao W, Alonso OF, et al. Uncoupling of local cerebral glucose metabolism and blood flow after acute fluid-percussion injury in rats. Am J Physiol 1997;272(6 Pt 2):H2859–68.

52. Hovda DA. Metabolic dysfunction. In: Narayan RK, Wilberger JE, Povlishock JT, editors. Neurotrauma. New York: McGraw-Hill; 1996. p. 1459–78.
53. Moore AH, Osteen CL, Chatziioannou AF, et al. Quantitative assessment of longitudinal metabolic changes in vivo after traumatic brain injury in the adult rat using FDG-microPET. J Cereb Blood Flow Metab 2000;20(10):1492–501.
54. Thoenen. Neurotrophins and neuronal plasticity. Science 1995;270(5236): 593–8.
55. Zafra F, Lindholm D, Castren E, et al. Regulation of brain-derived neurotrophic factor and nerve growth factor mRNA in primary cultures of hippocampal neurons and astrocytes. J Neurosci 1992;12(12):4793–9.
56. Tyler WJ, Pozzo-Miller LD. BDNF enhances quantal neurotransmitter release and increases the number of docked vesicles at the active zones of hippocampal excitatory synapses. J Neurosci 2001;21(12):4249–58.
57. Lessmann V, Gottmann K, Heumann R. BDNF and NT-4/5 enhance glutamatergic synaptic transmission in cultured hippocampal neurones. Neuroreport 1994; 6(1):21–5.
58. Levine ES, Dreyfus CF, Black IB, et al. Brain-derived neurotrophic factor rapidly enhances synaptic transmission in hippocampal neurons via postsynaptic tyrosine kinase receptors. Proc Natl Acad Sci U S A 1995;92(17):8074–7.
59. Takei N, Sasaoka K, Inoue K, et al. Brain-derived neurotrophic factor increases the stimulation-evoked release of glutamate and the levels of exocytosis-associated proteins in cultured cortical neurons from embryonic rats. J Neurochem 1997;68(1):370–5.
60. Neeper SA, Gomez-Pinilla F, Choi J, et al. Exercise and brain neurotrophins. Nature 1995;373(6510):109.
61. Griesbach GS, Hovda DA, Molteni R, et al. Voluntary exercise following traumatic brain injury: brain-derived neurotrophic factor upregulation and recovery of function. Neuroscience 2004;125(1):129–39.
62. Ip EY, Zanier ER, Moore AH, et al. Metabolic, neurochemical, and histologic responses to vibrissa motor cortex stimulation after traumatic brain injury. J Cereb Blood Flow Metab 2003;23(8):900–10.
63. Prins ML, Lee SM, Cheng CL, et al. Fluid percussion brain injury in the developing and adult rat: a comparative study of mortality, morphology, intracranial pressure and mean arterial blood pressure. Brain Res Dev Brain Res 1996; 95(2):272–82.
64. Thomas S, Prins ML, Samii M, et al. Cerebral metabolic response to traumatic brain injury sustained early in development: a 2-deoxy-D-glucose autoradiographic study. J Neurotrauma 2000;17(8):649–65.
65. McEwen BS. Stress and hippocampal plasticity. Annu Rev Neurosci 1999;22: 105–22.
66. McEwen BS, Magarinos AM. Stress and hippocampal plasticity: implications for the pathophysiology of affective disorders. Hum Psychopharmacol 2001;16(S1):S7–19.
67. Griesbach GS, Hovda DA, Tio DL, et al. Heightening of the stress response during the first weeks after a mild traumatic brain injury. Neuroscience 2011; 178:147–58.
68. Avital A, Richter-Levin G. Exposure to juvenile stress exacerbates the behavioural consequences of exposure to stress in the adult rat. Int J Neuropsychopharmacol 2005;8(2):163–73.
69. Pryce CR, Ruedi-Bettschen D, Dettling AC, et al. Long-term effects of early-life environmental manipulations in rodents and primates: potential animal models in depression research. Neurosci Biobehav Rev 2005;29(4-5):649–74.

70. Meaney MJ. Maternal care, gene expression, and the transmission of individual differences in stress reactivity across generations. Annu Rev Neurosci 2001;24: 1161–92.
71. Grundy PL, Harbuz MS, Jessop DS, et al. The hypothalamo-pituitary-adrenal axis response to experimental traumatic brain injury. J Neurotrauma 2001; 18(12):1373–81.
72. Roe SY, McGowan EM, Rothwell NJ. Evidence for the involvement of corticotrophin-releasing hormone in the pathogenesis of traumatic brain injury. Eur J Neurosci 1998;10(2):553–9.
73. Taylor AN, Rahman SU, Sanders NC, et al. Injury severity differentially affects short- and long-term neuroendocrine outcomes of traumatic brain injury. J Neurotrauma 2008;25(4):311–23.
74. Shohami E, Bass R, Trembovler V, et al. The effect of the adrenocortical axis upon recovery from closed head injury. J Neurotrauma 1995;12(6):1069–77.
75. Bergsneider M, Hovda DA, McArthur DL, et al. Metabolic recovery following human traumatic brain injury based on FDG-PET: time course and relationship to neurological disability. J Head Trauma Rehabil 2001;16(2):135–48.
76. McAllister TW, Flashman LA, McDonald BC, et al. Mechanisms of working memory dysfunction after mild and moderate TBI: evidence from functional MRI and neurogenetics. J Neurotrauma 2006;23(10):1450–67.
77. Bazarian JJ, Blyth B, Cimpello L. Bench to bedside: evidence for brain injury after concussion–looking beyond the computed tomography scan. Acad Emerg Med 2006;13(2):199–214.
78. Niogi SN, Mukherjee P, Ghajar J, et al. Extent of microstructural white matter injury in postconcussive syndrome correlates with impaired cognitive reaction time: a 3T diffusion tensor imaging study of mild traumatic brain injury. AJNR Am J Neuroradiol 2008;29(5):967–73.
79. Johnson JA. The hypothalamic-pituitary-adrenal axis in critical illness. AACN Clin Issues 2006;17(1):39–49.
80. Woolf PD, Cox C, Kelly M, et al. The adrenocortical response to brain injury: correlation with the severity of neurologic dysfunction, effects of intoxication, and patient outcome. Alcohol Clin Exp Res 1990;14(6):917–21.
81. Steinbok P, Thompson G. Serum cortisol abnormalities after craniocerebral trauma. Neurosurgery 1979;5(5):559–65.
82. Cernak I, Savic VJ, Lazarov A, et al. Neuroendocrine responses following graded traumatic brain injury in male adults. Brain Inj 1999;13(12):1005–15.
83. Cohan P, Wang C, McArthur DL, et al. Acute secondary adrenal insufficiency after traumatic brain injury: a prospective study. Crit Care Med 2005;33(10):2358–66.
84. Bondanelli M, De Marinis L, Ambrosio MR, et al. Occurrence of pituitary dysfunction following traumatic brain injury. J Neurotrauma 2004;21(6):685–96.
85. Niederland T, Makovi H, Gal V, et al. Abnormalities of pituitary function after traumatic brain injury in children. J Neurotrauma 2007;24(1):119–27.
86. Falkenberg T, Mohammed AK, Henriksson B, et al. Increased expression of brain-derived neurotrophic factor mRNA in rat hippocampus is associated with improved spatial memory and enriched environment. Neurosci Lett 1992;138:153–6.
87. Kesslak JP, So V, Choi J, et al. Learning upregulates brain-derived neurotrophic factor messenger ribonucleic acid: a mechanism to facilitate encoding and circuit maintenance? Behav Neurosci 1998;112(4):1012–9.
88. Diamond MC, Lindner B, Raymond A. Extensive cortical depth measurements and neuron size increase in the cortex of environmentally enriched rats. J Comp Neurol 1967;131:357–64.

89. Rosenzweig MR, Krech D, Bennett EL, et al. Effects of environmental complexity and training on brain chemistry and anatomy: a replication and extension. J Comp Physiol Psychol 1962;55:429–37.

90. Diamond MC, Krech D, Rosenzweig MR. The effects of an enriched environment on the histology of the rat cerebral cortex. J Comp Neurol 1964;123:111–20.

91. Fineman I, Giza CC, Nahed BV, et al. Inhibition of neocortical plasticity during development by a moderate concussive brain injury. J Neurotrauma 2000; 17(9):739–49.

92. Ip EY, Giza CC, Griesbach GS, et al. Effects of enriched environment and fluid percussion injury on dendritic arborization within the cerebral cortex of the developing rat. J Neurotrauma 2002;19(5):573–85.

93. Giza CC, Griesbach GS, Hovda DA. Experience-dependent behavioral plasticity is disturbed following traumatic injury to the immature brain. Behav Brain Res 2005;157(1):11–22.

94. Gurkoff GG, Giza CC, Hovda DA. Lateral fluid percussion injury in the developing rat causes an acute, mild behavioral dysfunction in the absence of significant cell death. Brain Res 2006;1077(1):24–36.

95. Giza CC, Maria NS, Hovda DA. N-Methyl-D-aspartate receptor subunit changes after traumatic injury to the developing brain. J Neurotrauma 2006;23(6):950–61.

96. Hellmich HL, Garcia JM, Shimamura M, et al. Traumatic brain injury and hemorrhagic hypotension suppress neuroprotective gene expression in injured hippocampal neurons. Anesthesiology 2005;102:806–14.

97. Hicks RR, Li C, Zhang L, et al. Alterations in BDNF and trkB mRNA levels in the cerebral cortex following experimental brain trauma in rats. J Neurotrauma 1999;16(6):501–10.

98. Yang K, Perez-Polo JR, Mu XS, et al. Increased expression of brain-derived neurotrophic factor but not neurotrophin-3 mRNA in rat brain after cortical impact injury. J Neurosci Res 1996;44(2):157–64.

99. Oyesiku NM, Evans CO, Houston S, et al. Regional changes in the expression of neurotrophic factors and their receptors following acute traumatic brain injury in the adult rat brain. Brain Res 1999;833(2):161–72.

100. Schoups AA, Elliott RC, Friedman WJ, et al. NGF and BDNF are differentially modulated by visual experience in the developing geniculocortical pathway. Brain Res Dev Brain Res 1995;86(1-2):326–34.

101. Zhou J, Pliego-Rivero B, Bradford HF, et al. The BDNF content of postnatal and adult rat brain: the effects of 6-hydroxydopamine lesions in adult brain. Brain Res Dev Brain Res 1996;97(2):297–303.

102. Lein ES, Shatz CJ. Rapid regulation of brain-derived neurotrophic factor mRNA within eye-specific circuits during ocular dominance column formation. J Neurosci 2000;20(4):1470–83.

103. Griesbach GS, Gomez-Pinilla F, Hovda DA. The upregulation of plasticity-related proteins following TBI is disrupted with acute voluntary exercise. Brain Res 2004;1016(2):154–62.

104. Griesbach GS, Hovda DA, Molteni R, et al. Alterations in BDNF and synapsin I within the occipital cortex and hippocampus after mild traumatic brain injury in the developing rat: reflections of injury-induced neuroplasticity. J Neurotrauma 2002;19(7):803–14.

105. Dancause N, Barbay S, Frost SB, et al. Extensive cortical rewiring after brain injury. J Neurosci 2005;25(44):10167–79.

106. Stein DG, Hoffman SW. Concepts of CNS plasticity in the context of brain damage and repair. J Head Trauma Rehabil 2003;18(4):317–41.

107. Desmurget M, Bonnetblanc F, Duffau H. Contrasting acute and slow-growing lesions: a new door to brain plasticity. Brain 2007;130(Pt 4):898–914.
108. Dunn-Meynell AA, Levin BE. Lateralized effect of unilateral somatosensory cortex contusion on behavior and cortical reorganization. Brain Res 1995; 675(1-2):143–56.
109. Jansen EM, Low WC. Quantitative analysis of contralateral hemisphere hypertrophy and sensorimotor performance in adult rats following unilateral neonatal ischemic-hypoxic brain injury. Brain Res 1996;708(1-2):93–9.
110. Kozlowski D, Schallert T. Relationship between dendritic pruning and behavioral recovery following sensorimotor cortex lesions. Behav Brain Res 1998;97:89–98.
111. Florence SL, Taub HB, Kaas JH. Large-scale sprouting of cortical connections after peripheral injury in adult macaque monkeys. Science 1998;282(5391):1117–21.
112. Burek MJ, Oppenheim RW. Programmed cell death in the developing nervous system. Brain Pathol 1996;6(4):427–46.
113. Catsicas S, Thanos S, Clarke PG. Major role for neuronal death during brain development: refinement of topographical connections. Proc Natl Acad Sci U S A 1987;84(22):8165–8.
114. Adelson PD, Dixon CE, Kochanek PM. Long-term dysfunction following diffuse traumatic brain injury in the immature rat. J Neurotrauma 2000;17(4):273–82.
115. Anderson V, Catroppa C, Morse S, et al. Functional plasticity or vulnerability after early brain injury? Pediatrics 2005;116(6):1374–82.
116. Levin HS, Eisenberg HM, Wigg NR, et al. Memory and intellectual ability after head injury in children and adolescents. Neurosurgery 1982;11(5):668–73.
117. Chapman SB, Levin HS, Wanek A, et al. Discourse after closed head injury in young children. Brain Lang 1998;61(3):420–49.
118. Klonoff H, Low MD, Clark C. Head injuries in children: a prospective five year follow-up. J Neurol Neurosurg Psychiatry 1977;40(12):1211–9.
119. Johnson MH. Sensitive periods in functional brain development: problems and prospects. Dev Psychobiol 2005;46(3):287–92.
120. Giza CC, Prins ML. Is being plastic fantastic? Mechanisms of altered plasticity after developmental traumatic brain injury. Dev Neurosci 2006;28(4-5):364–79.
121. Jacobs R, Harvey AS, Anderson V. Executive function following focal frontal lobe lesions: impact of timing of lesion on outcome. Cortex 2007;43(6):792–805.
122. Anderson V, Catroppa C. Memory outcome at 5 years post-childhood traumatic brain injury. Brain Inj 2007;21(13-14):1399–409.
123. Anderson V, Spencer-Smith M, Coleman L, et al. Children's executive functions: are they poorer after very early brain insult. Neuropsychologia 2010;48(7): 2041–50.
124. Anderson V, Brown S, Newitt H, et al. Long-term outcome from childhood traumatic brain injury: intellectual ability, personality, and quality of life. Neuropsychology 2011;25(2):176–84.
125. Gomez-Pinilla F, Dao L, So V. Physical exercise induces FGF-2 and its mRNA in the hippocampus. Brain Res 1997;764(1-2):1–8.
126. Carro E, Trejo JL, Busiguina S, et al. Circulating insulin-like growth factor I mediates the protective effects of physical exercise against brain insults of different etiology and anatomy. J Neurosci 2001;21(15):5678–84.
127. van Praag H, Kempermann G, Gage FH. Running increases cell proliferation and neurogenesis in the adult mouse dentate gyrus. Nat Neurosci 1999;2(3): 266–70.
128. Cotman CW, Berchtold NC. Exercise: a behavioral intervention to enhance brain health and plasticity. Trends Neurosci 2002;25(6):295–301.

129. Fabel K, Tam B, Kaufer D, et al. VEGF is necessary for exercise-induced adult hippocampal neurogenesis. Eur J Neurosci 2003;18(10):2803–12.

130. van Praag H, Shubert T, Zhao C, et al. Exercise enhances learning and hippocampal neurogenesis in aged mice. J Neurosci 2005;25(38):8680–5.

131. Kleim JA, Jones TA, Schallert T. Motor enrichment and the induction of plasticity before or after brain injury. Neurochem Res 2003;28(11):1757–69.

132. Kolb B. Synaptic plasticity and the organization of behaviour after early and late brain injury. Can J Exp Psychol 1999;53(1):62–76.

133. Ivanco TL, Greenough WT. Physiological consequences of morphologically detectable synaptic plasticity: potential uses for examining recovery following damage. Neuropharmacology 2000;39(5):765–76.

134. Albensi BC. Models of brain injury and alterations in synaptic plasticity. J Neurosci Res 2001;65(4):279–83.

135. Griesbach GS, Hovda DA, Gomez-Pinilla F. Exercise-induced improvement in cognitive performance after traumatic brain injury in rats is dependent on BDNF activation. Brain Res 2009;1288:105–15.

136. Dishman RK, Berthoud HR, Booth FW, et al. Neurobiology of exercise. Obesity (Silver Spring) 2006;14(3):345–56.

137. Griesbach GS, Gomez-Pinilla F, Hovda DA. Time window for voluntary exercise-induced increases in hippocampal neuroplasticity molecules after traumatic brain injury is severity dependent. J Neurotrauma 2007;24(7):1161–71.

138. Smith MA, Makino S, Kvetnansky R, et al. Effects of stress on neurotrophic factor expression in the rat brain. Ann N Y Acad Sci 1995;771:234–9.

139. Hansson AC, Sommer WH, Metsis M, et al. Corticosterone actions on the hippocampal brain-derived neurotrophic factor expression are mediated by exon IV promoter. J Neuroendocrinol 2006;18(2):104–14.

140. Gronli J, Bramham C, Murison R, et al. Chronic mild stress inhibits BDNF protein expression and CREB activation in the dentate gyrus but not in the hippocampus proper. Pharmacol Biochem Behav 2006;85(4):842–9.

141. Hansson AC, Cintra A, Belluardo N, et al. Gluco- and mineralocorticoid receptor-mediated regulation of neurotrophic factor gene expression in the dorsal hippocampus and the neocortex of the rat. Eur J Neurosci 2000;12(8):2918–34.

142. Schaaf MJ, De Kloet ER, Vreugdenhil E. Corticosterone effects on BDNF expression in the hippocampus. Implications for memory formation. Stress 2000;3(3):201–8.

143. Dishman RK, Renner KJ, White-Welkley JE, et al. Treadmill exercise training augments brain norepinephrine response to familiar and novel stress. Brain Res Bull 2000;52(5):337–42.

144. Dalsgaard MK, Volianitis S, Yoshiga CC, et al. Cerebral metabolism during upper and lower body exercise. J Appl Physiol 2004;97(5):1733–9.

145. Smith PJ, Blumenthal JA, Hoffman BM, et al. Aerobic exercise and neurocognitive performance: a meta-analytic review of randomized controlled trials. Psychosom Med 2010;72(3):239–52.

146. Hillman CH, Erickson KI, Kramer AF. Be smart, exercise your heart: exercise effects on brain and cognition. Nat Rev Neurosci 2008;9(1):58–65.

147. Wipfli BM, Rethorst CD, Landers DM. The anxiolytic effects of exercise: a meta-analysis of randomized trials and dose-response analysis. J Sport Exerc Psychol 2008;30(4):392–410.

148. Smits JA, Berry AC, Rosenfield D, et al. Reducing anxiety sensitivity with exercise. Depress Anxiety 2008;25(8):689–99.

149. Merom D, Phongsavan P, Wagner R, et al. Promoting walking as an adjunct intervention to group cognitive behavioral therapy for anxiety disorders–a pilot group randomized trial. J Anxiety Disord 2008;22(6):959–68.
150. Castelli DM, Hillman CH, Buck SM, et al. Physical fitness and academic achievement in third- and fifth-grade students. J Sport Exerc Psychol 2007; 29(2):239–52.
151. Chaddock L, Hillman CH, Buck SM, et al. Aerobic fitness and executive control of relational memory in preadolescent children. Med Sci Sports Exerc 2011; 43(2):344–9.
152. Hillman CH, Pontifex MB, Raine LB, et al. The effect of acute treadmill walking on cognitive control and academic achievement in preadolescent children. Neuroscience 2009;159(3):1044–54.
153. Davis CL, Tomporowski PD, Boyle CA, et al. Effects of aerobic exercise on overweight children's cognitive functioning: a randomized controlled trial. Res Q Exerc Sport 2007;78(5):510–9.
154. Koseoglu E, Akboyraz A, Soyuer A, et al. Aerobic exercise and plasma beta endorphin levels in patients with migrainous headache without aura. Cephalalgia 2003;23(10):972–6.
155. Lockett DM, Campbell JF. The effects of aerobic exercise on migraine. Headache 1992;32(1):50–4.
156. Gordon WA, Sliwinski M, Echo J, et al. The benefits of exercise in individuals with traumatic brain injury: a retrospective study. J Head Trauma Rehabil 1998;13(4):58–67.
157. Ashman TA, Gordon WA, Cantor JB, et al. Neurobehavioral consequences of traumatic brain injury. Mt Sinai J Med 2006;73(7):999–1005.
158. Bombardier CH, Fann JR, Temkin NR, et al. Rates of major depressive disorder and clinical outcomes following traumatic brain injury. JAMA 2010;303(19): 1938–45.
159. Driver S, O'connor J, Lox C, et al. Evaluation of an aquatics programme on fitness parameters of individuals with a brain injury. Brain Inj 2004;18(9): 847–59.
160. Ekeland E, Heian F, Hagen KB, et al. Exercise to improve self-esteem in children and young people. Cochrane Database Syst Rev 2004;1:CD003683.
161. Gagnon I, Galli C, Friedman D, et al. Active rehabilitation for children who are slow to recover following sport-related concussion. Brain Inj 2009;23(12): 956–64.
162. Majerske CW, Mihalik JP, Ren D, et al. Concussion in sports: postconcussive activity levels, symptoms, and neurocognitive performance. J Athl Train 2008; 43(3):265–74.
163. Laurer HL, Bareyre FM, Lee VM, et al. Mild head injury increasing the brain's vulnerability to a second concussive impact. J Neurosurg 2001;95(5):859–70.
164. Schulz MR, Marshall SW, Mueller FO, et al. Incidence and risk factors for concussion in high school athletes, North Carolina, 1996–1999. Am J Epidemiol 2004;160(10):937–44.
165. Aubry M, Cantu R, Dvorak J, et al. Summary and agreement statement of the First International Conference on Concussion in Sport, Vienna 2001. Recommendations for the improvement of safety and health of athletes who may suffer concussive injuries. Br J Sports Med 2002;36(1):6–10.
166. Weightman MM, Bolgla R, McCulloch KL, et al. Physical therapy recommendations for service members with mild traumatic brain injury. J Head Trauma Rehabil 2010;25(3):206–18.

167. McCrory P, Meeuwisse W, Johnston K, et al. Consensus Statement on Concussion in Sport: the 3rd International Conference on Concussion in Sport held in Zurich, November 2008. Br J Sports Med 2009;43(Suppl 1):i76–90.
168. Field AS, Hasan K, Jellison BJ, et al. Diffusion tensor imaging in an infant with traumatic brain swelling. AJNR Am J Neuroradiol 2003;24(7):1461–4.
169. Vagnozzi R, Signoretti S, Cristofori L, et al. Assessment of metabolic brain damage and recovery following mild traumatic brain injury: a multicentre, proton magnetic resonance spectroscopic study in concussed patients. Brain 2010; 133(11):3232–42.
170. Pettus EH, Povlishock JT. Characterization of a distinct set of intra-axonal ultrastructural changes associated with traumatically induced alteration in axolemmal permeability. Brain Res 1996;722(1-2):1–11.
171. Povlishock JT, Christman CW. The pathobiology of traumatically induced axonal injury in animals and humans: a review of current thoughts. J Neurotrauma 1995; 12(4):555–64.
172. Buki A, Povlishock JT. All roads lead to disconnection? Traumatic axonal injury revisited. Acta Neurochir (Wien) 2006;148(2):181–93.
173. Reeves TM, Phillips LL, Povlishock JT. Myelinated and unmyelinated axons of the corpus callosum differ in vulnerability and functional recovery following traumatic brain injury. Exp Neurol 2005;196(1):126–37.
174. Mac Donald CL, Dikranian K, Bayly P, et al. Diffusion tensor imaging reliably detects experimental traumatic axonal injury and indicates approximate time of injury. J Neurosci 2007;27(44):11869–76.
175. Mac Donald CL, Dikranian K, Song SK, et al. Detection of traumatic axonal injury with diffusion tensor imaging in a mouse model of traumatic brain injury. Exp Neurol 2007;205(1):116–31.
176. Adams JH, Graham DI, Murray LS, et al. Diffuse axonal injury due to nonmissile head injury in humans: an analysis of 45 cases. Ann Neurol 1982; 12(6):557–63.
177. Adams JH, Jennett B, Murray LS, et al. Neuropathological findings in disabled survivors of a head injury. J Neurotrauma 2011;28(5):701–9.
178. Blumbergs PC, Scott G, Manavis J, et al. Staining of amyloid precursor protein to study axonal damage in mild head injury. Lancet 1994;344(8929): 1055–6.
179. Blumbergs PC, Scott G, Manavis J, et al. Topography of axonal injury as defined by amyloid precursor protein and the sector scoring method in mild and severe closed head injury. J Neurotrauma 1995;12(4):565–72.
180. Wozniak JR, Krach L, Ward E, et al. Neurocognitive and neuroimaging correlates of pediatric traumatic brain injury: a diffusion tensor imaging (DTI) study. Arch Clin Neuropsychol 2007;22(5):555–68.
181. Oni MB, Wilde EA, Bigler ED, et al. Diffusion tensor imaging analysis of frontal lobes in pediatric traumatic brain injury. J Child Neurol 2010;25(8):976–84.
182. Wilde EA, McCauley SR, Hunter JV, et al. Diffusion tensor imaging of acute mild traumatic brain injury in adolescents. Neurology 2008;70(12):948–55.
183. Huang M, Theilmann RJ, Robb A, et al. Integrated imaging approach with MEG and DTI to detect mild traumatic brain injury in military and civilian patients. J Neurotrauma 2009;26(8):1213–26.
184. Babikian T, Tong KA, Galloway NR, et al. Diffusion-weighted imaging predicts cognition in pediatric brain injury. Pediatr Neurol 2009;41(6):406–12.
185. Niogi SN, Mukherjee P. Diffusion tensor imaging of mild traumatic brain injury. J Head Trauma Rehabil 2010;25(4):241–55.

186. McKee AC, Cantu RC, Nowinski CJ, et al. Chronic traumatic encephalopathy in athletes: progressive tauopathy after repetitive head injury. J Neuropathol Exp Neurol 2009;68(7):709–35.
187. Iwata A, Chen XH, McIntosh TK, et al. Long-term accumulation of amyloid-beta in axons following brain trauma without persistent upregulation of amyloid precursor protein genes. J Neuropathol Exp Neurol 2002;61(12):1056–68.
188. Blasko I, Beer R, Bigl M, et al. Experimental traumatic brain injury in rats stimulates the expression, production and activity of Alzheimer's disease beta-secretase (BACE-1). J Neural Transm 2004;111(4):523–36.
189. Cribbs DH, Chen LS, Cotman CW, et al. Injury induces presenilin-1 gene expression in mouse brain. Neuroreport 1996;7(11):1773–6.
190. Smith DH, Nakamura M, McIntosh TK, et al. Brain trauma induces massive hippocampal neuron death linked to a surge in beta-amyloid levels in mice over-expressing mutant amyloid precursor protein. Am J Pathol 1998;153(3): 1005–10.
191. Uryu K, Laurer H, McIntosh T, et al. Repetitive mild brain trauma accelerates Abeta deposition, lipid peroxidation, and cognitive impairment in a transgenic mouse model of Alzheimer amyloidosis. J Neurosci 2002;22(2):446–54.
192. Loane DJ, Pocivavsek A, Moussa CE, et al. Amyloid precursor protein secretases as therapeutic targets for traumatic brain injury. Nat Med 2009;15(4): 377–9.
193. Chen XH, Siman R, Iwata A, et al. Long-term accumulation of amyloid-beta, beta-secretase, presenilin-1, and caspase-3 in damaged axons following brain trauma. Am J Pathol 2004;165(2):357–71.
194. Magnoni S, Brody DL. New perspectives on amyloid-beta dynamics after acute brain injury: moving between experimental approaches and studies in the human brain. Arch Neurol 2010;67(9):1068–73.
195. Bogdanoff B, Natter HM. Incidence of cavum septum pellucidum in adults: a sign of boxer's encephalopathy. Neurology 1989;39(7):991–2.
196. Silbert PL, Gubbay SS, Vaughan RJ. Cavum septum pellucidum and obstructive hydrocephalus. J Neurol Neurosurg Psychiatry 1993;56(7):820–2.
197. McKee AC, Gavett BE, Stern RA, et al. TDP-43 proteinopathy and motor neuron disease in chronic traumatic encephalopathy. J Neuropathol Exp Neurol 2010; 69(9):918–29.
198. Strich SJ. Diffuse degeneration of the cerebral white matter in severe dementia following head injury. J Neurol Neurosurg Psychiatry 1956;19(3):163–85.
199. Gale SD, Burr RB, Bigler ED, et al. Fornix degeneration and memory in traumatic brain injury. Brain Res Bull 1993;32(4):345–9.
200. Binder LI, Guillozet-Bongaarts AL, Garcia-Sierra F, et al. Tau, tangles, and Alzheimer's disease. Biochim Biophys Acta 2005;1739(2-3):216–23.
201. Serbest G, Burkhardt MF, Siman R, et al. Temporal profiles of cytoskeletal protein loss following traumatic axonal injury in mice. Neurochem Res 2007; 32(12):2006–14.
202. Hof PR, Bouras C, Buee L, et al. Differential distribution of neurofibrillary tangles in the cerebral cortex of dementia pugilistica and Alzheimer's disease cases. Acta Neuropathol 1992;85(1):23–30.
203. Geddes JF, Vowles GH, Nicoll JA, et al. Neuronal cytoskeletal changes are an early consequence of repetitive head injury. Acta Neuropathol 1999;98(2):171–8.
204. Omalu B, Bailes J, Hamilton RL, et al. Emerging histomorphologic phenotypes of chronic traumatic encephalopathy (CTE) in American athletes. Neurosurgery 2011;69(1):173–83.

205. Frost B, Jacks RL, Diamond MI. Propagation of tau misfolding from the outside to the inside of a cell. J Biol Chem 2009;284(19):12845–52.
206. Johnson VE, Stewart W, Smith DH. Traumatic brain injury and amyloid-beta pathology: a link to Alzheimer's disease? Nat Rev Neurosci 2010;11(5):361–70.
207. Chen XH, Johnson VE, Uryu K, et al. A lack of amyloid beta plaques despite persistent accumulation of amyloid beta in axons of long-term survivors of traumatic brain injury. Brain Pathol 2009;19(2):214–23.
208. Appel SH, Cwik VA, Day JW. Trauma, TDP-43, and amyotrophic lateral sclerosis. Muscle Nerve 2010;42(6):851–2.
209. Armon C, Miller RG. Correspondence regarding: TDP-43 proteinopathy and motor neuron disease in chronic traumatic encephalopathy. J Neuropathol Exp Neurol 2010:69;918-29. J Neuropathol Exp Neurol 2011;70(1):97–8 [author reply: 98–100].
210. Zetterberg H, Hietala MA, Jonsson M, et al. Neurochemical aftermath of amateur boxing. Arch Neurol 2006;63(9):1277–80.
211. Zetterberg H, Tanriverdi F, Unluhizarci K, et al. Sustained release of neuron-specific enolase to serum in amateur boxers. Brain Inj 2009;23(9):723–6.
212. Saunders AM, Strittmatter WJ, Schmechel D, et al. Association of apolipoprotein E allele epsilon 4 with late-onset familial and sporadic Alzheimer's disease. Neurology 1993;43(8):1467–72.
213. Corder EH, Saunders AM, Strittmatter WJ, et al. Gene dose of apolipoprotein E type 4 allele and the risk of Alzheimer's disease in late onset families. Science 1993;261(5123):921–3.
214. Strittmatter WJ, Saunders AM, Schmechel D, et al. Apolipoprotein E: high-avidity binding to beta-amyloid and increased frequency of type 4 allele in late-onset familial Alzheimer disease. Proc Natl Acad Sci U S A 1993;90(5):1977–81.
215. Jordan BD. Chronic traumatic brain injury associated with boxing. Semin Neurol 2000;20(2):179–85.
216. Jordan BD, Relkin NR, Ravdin LD, et al. Apolipoprotein E epsilon4 associated with chronic traumatic brain injury in boxing. JAMA 1997;278(2):136–40.
217. Corder EH, Saunders AM, Risch NJ, et al. Protective effect of apolipoprotein E type 2 allele for late onset Alzheimer disease. Nat Genet 1994;7(2):180–4.

Sport-Related Concussion: On-Field and Sideline Assessment

Kevin M. Guskiewicz, PhD, ATC[a],*, Steven P. Broglio, PhD, ATC[b]

KEYWORDS

- Mild traumatic brain injury • Symptom assessment
- Balance and postural control • Neuropsychological function
- Emergency action plan

The careful and well-planned sideline assessment of concussion can be the difference between a good and bad outcome when managing sport-related concussion. In most cases, the sideline assessment serves as a triage for determining if an injury, such as a concussion, has actually occurred, and if so, establishes a benchmark for determining whether a more serious and potentially catastrophic condition could be developing. Given its description as "a complex pathophysiological process affecting the brain, induced by traumatic biomechanical forces,"[1,2] concussions can evolve into something more serious if signs and symptoms go undetected or are ignored. Although these are very rare events, they must always be at the forefront of the clinician's mind.

Concussions occur in all sports, and though the incidence varies widely between sports,[3] in some sports (eg, women's ice hockey) the incidence of concussion may exceed that of all other injuries.[4] Regardless of the setting, sports medicine clinicians must be prepared to manage these complex and somewhat misunderstood injuries, which have been labeled by the Centers for Disease Control and Prevention as a "hidden epidemic." Developing and instituting a concussion policy and management protocol constitutes the first step in properly treating the athlete suspected of sustaining a concussion, which should be backed by proper planning and practice of the on-field management strategy.

Much of the inherent complexity in evaluating athletes suspected of sustaining a concussion lies in the broad spectrum of outcomes associated with the injury. Knowing the athlete and his or her background, concussion history, and ability and

[a] Department of Exercise and Sport Science, University of North Carolina, 209 Fetzer Hall, CB#8700, South Road, Chapel Hill, NC 27599-8700, USA
[b] School of Kinesiology, University of Michigan, 3736 CCRB, Central Campus Recreation Building, 401 Washenaw Avenue, Ann Arbor, MI 48109, USA
* Corresponding author.
E-mail address: gus@email.unc.edu

Phys Med Rehabil Clin N Am 22 (2011) 603–617
doi:10.1016/j.pmr.2011.08.003
1047-9651/11/$ – see front matter © 2011 Elsevier Inc. All rights reserved.

pmr.theclinics.com

willingness to provide information about his or her condition can minimize the challenges of evaluating the injury. Research has shown that impact location and magnitude,[5,6] previous history of concussive injuries,[7] learning disabilities,[8] and age[9] can alter the risk of concussion and in some cases the outcomes following injury. To further complicate matters, no definitive diagnostic tool is available for concussion at this time. Standard computed tomography and magnetic resonance imaging (MRI) are insensitive to the functional deficits observed following concussion. Functional MRI, diffuse tensor imaging, single-photon emission computed tomography, and magnetic resonance spectroscopy are showing promise, but their widespread use as an objective diagnostic tool has not yet been substantiated. Several objective clinical measures (neuropsychological and balance tests) are recommended to support the clinical examination. Although these tools have vastly improved the concussion diagnosis in recent years, the clinical examination remains the gold standard for evaluation.[10]

EMERGENCY ACTION PLANNING AND ESTABLISHING A CONCUSSION POLICY

Before the first preseason practice, the sports medicine clinician in charge of on-field injury management should make sure to have an emergency action plan in place. This plan should incorporate strategies to address heat illness, cardiac sudden death, weather and, of course, a specific plan for managing concussion and cervical spine injury (**Box 1**). When developing the concussion component of the plan, the clinician should develop a concussion policy and concussion protocol. The protocol is different from the policy, in that it specifically outlines the clinical tests that will be used for assessments and a graduated return-to-play progression. The policy itself outlines the steps to be put in place preseason, including roles and responsibilities of the team. The policy should at the very least consider 4 components: (1) preseason planning, (2) on-field/sideline evaluation, (3) removal from play, and (4) graduated return-to-play progression. Concussion education materials and sample concussion policies are available at http://www.ncaa.org/health-safety. Although the focus of this article is on the sideline examination and removal from play, the planning component is very important. It is during the preseason planning and practice that the roles and responsibilities in the event of a concussion should be clarified. For example, the concussion protocol should ensure clarity and an understanding regarding:

- Who will be responsible for the on-field response?
- Who will conduct the emergency assessment and handle communication if advanced help is needed?
- Who will observe the athlete on the sideline following injury?
- Who will make a concussion diagnosis or return-to-play decision, especially in the absence of a physician?
- Who will communicate the diagnosis and prognosis with the parents and coaches?

In addition, preseason planning should include drills and planning for sporting events both at the home venue and outside of the local area. In both of these situations, it is important to assess the availability of emergency medical responders and the location of trauma centers, when available.

Depending on the setting (youth, high school, college, or professional), the sports medicine team should develop a plan for educating all personnel about concussion to include athletes, parents, coaches, and league and school officials. The education program should make it clear that it is the responsibility of the athletes, parents, and coaches to report any symptoms of concussion to the medical staff. The program should also discuss the potential long-term consequences of concussion, and expectations for safe play.

Ideally the concussion policy and protocol will include a preseason baseline evaluation, including a clinical examination that evaluates concussion-related symptoms, and the athlete's orientation, memory, concentration, and balance. In addition, baseline neuropsychological testing has been shown to be a helpful adjunct and can be readministered post injury to identify the effects of the injury. The most commonly used neuropsychological tests assess a range of brain behaviors including memory, concentration, information processing, executive function, and reaction time. In some instances additional health care professionals may be needed to administer and interpret these tests.

KNOW YOUR ATHLETES AND ENSURE THEY UNDERSTAND CONCUSSION

In many settings, athletic trainers represent the front line of defense in protecting concussed athletes from returning to a game or practice and placing themselves at risk for further injury. Athletic trainers have the advantage of knowing the personalities and habits of their athletes, which affords them the opportunity to rapidly identify alterations that would lead one to suspect a concussion has occurred. Once an athlete is suspected of sustaining a concussion, a physician should be involved in the return-to-play decision. Because the athletic trainer is often the lone health care provider, establishing an agreed-upon concussion policy and protocol beforehand is very important for appropriate management. Regardless of the setting, the athletes, coaches, and medical personnel must be educated about concussion and should read and sign a statement confirming that they understand the signs and symptoms of a concussion, and understand their responsibility to report a suspected concussion to the team's medical staff (**Table 1**).

THE ON-FIELD/SIDELINE ASSESSMENT
Primary Survey

Identification of concussions remains a challenge for sports medicine clinicians, which underscores the importance of knowing athletes and their dispositions. Many athletes will hide symptoms of a concussion because they do not want to be removed from participation or let down their coach and teammates.[11] In most cases, the athlete will show no outwardly visible signs of concussion; in fact, only 9% to 10% of all concussions will involve a loss of consciousness.[7,12] In the event an athlete is rendered unconscious, the clinician should also suspect a cervical spine injury when approaching him or her on the playing field. Following a determination of level of consciousness, the initial assessment should include a primary survey of the athlete's airway, breathing, and circulation while maintaining the cervical spine in a neutral position. The primary survey can usually be completed in a matter of seconds to a few minutes. Once the athlete regains consciousness and more severe injuries such as cervical spine or cranial fractures have been ruled out, the athlete can be taken to the sideline for further evaluation. If the athlete remains in an unconscious state, he or she should be transported immediately to the nearest medical facility for further evaluation. Other considerations for physician referral following a suspected concussion are outlined in **Box 2**, but typically involve any indication of neurologic deterioration.

Secondary Survey

The clinician conducting the secondary survey on the sideline can benefit from the results of preseason baseline scores. The highly variable nature of concussion calls

Box 1
General guidelines for developing emergency action plans

1. Establish roles: adapt to specific team/sport/venue; it may be best to have more than one person assigned to each role in case of absence/turnover
   a. Immediate care of the athlete
      i. Typically physician, Certified Athletic Trainer, first responder, but also those trained in basic life support
   b. Activation of emergency medical system
      i. Could be school administrator, anyone
   c. Emergency equipment retrieval
      i. Could be student assistant, coach, anyone
   d. Direction of emergency medical responders to scene
      i. Could be administrator, coach, student assistant, anyone
2. Communication
   a. Primary method
      i. May be fixed (landline) or mobile (cellular phone, radio)
      ii. List all key personnel and all phones associated with this person
   b. Backup method
      i. Often a landline
   c. Test before event
      i. Cell phone/radio reception can vary, batteries charged, landline working
      ii. Make sure communication methods are accessible (identify and post location, are there locks or other barriers, change available for pay-phone)
   d. Activation of emergency medical system
      i. Identify contact numbers (911, ambulance, police, fire, hospital, poison control, suicide hotline)
      ii. Prepare script (caller name/location/phone number, nature of emergency, number of victims and their condition, what treatment initiated, specific directions to scene)
      iii. Post both of the above near communication devices, other visible locations in venue, and circulate to appropriate personnel
   e. Student emergency information
      i. Critical medical information (conditions, medications, allergies)
      ii. Emergency contact information (parent/guardian)
      iii. Accessible (keep with athletic trainer for example)
3. Emergency equipment
   a. Automated external defibrillators, bag-valve mask, spine board, splints
   b. Personnel trained in advance on proper use
   c. Must be accessible (identify and post location, within acceptable distance for each venue, are there locks or other barriers)
   d. Proper condition and maintenance
      i. document inspection (log book)

4. Emergency transportation

  a. Ambulance on site for high-risk events (know difference between basic life support and advanced life support vehicles/personnel)

    i. Designated location

    ii. Clear route for exiting venue

  b. When ambulance not on site

    i. Entrance to venue clearly marked and accessible

    ii. Identify parking/loading point and confirm area is clear

  c. Coordinate ahead of time with local emergency medical services

5. Additional considerations

  a. Must be venue specific (football field, gymnasium, and so forth)

  b. Put plan in writing

  c. Involve all appropriate personnel (administrators, coaches, sports medicine, emergency medical system)

    i. Development

    ii. Approval with signatures

  d. Post the plan in visible areas of each venue and distribute

  e. Review plan at least annually

  f. Rehearse plan at least annually

  g. Document

    i. Events of emergency situation

    ii. Evaluation of response

    iii. Rehearsal, training, equipment maintenance

Specific considerations for Head and Neck Injury:

1. Athletic trainer/first responder should be prepared to remove the face-mask from a football helmet to access a victim's airway without moving the cervical spine

2. Sports medicine team should communicate ahead of time with local emergency medical system

  a. Agree on cervical spine immobilization techniques (eg, leave helmet and shoulder pads on for football players)

  b. Type of immobilization equipment available on site and from emergency medical system

3. Athletes and coaches should be trained not to move victim

for an individualized approach to injury management[1,2] and warrants the use of base-line assessments for each athlete during an uninjured state. Regardless of the specific tests used, the evaluation should include measures of concussion-related symptoms, balance, and neuropsychological function.[13] Each of these are addressed in detail here. When evaluating an athlete following a suspected concussive blow, the premorbid data can be used to objectively identify postinjury change that will support the decision derived from the clinical examination.

The sideline assessment for concussion should follow a standardized protocol that involves the use of a 7-step process to include history, observation, palpation, special tests, range of motion (ROM) tests, strength tests, and functional tests. In many

---

Table 1
Student-athlete concussion statement

☐ I understand that it is my responsibility to report all injuries and illnesses to my athletic trainer and/or team physician.

☐ I have read and understand the *Concussion Fact Sheet.*

After reading the *Concussion Fact Sheet*, I am aware of the following information:

_____ A concussion is a brain injury, which I am responsible for reporting to my team physician or athletic trainer.

_____ A concussion can affect my ability to perform everyday activities, including reaction time, balance, sleep, and classroom performance.

_____I realize I cannot see a concussion, but I might notice some symptoms right away. Other symptoms can show up hours or days later.

_____ If I suspect a teammate has a concussion, I am responsible for reporting the injury to my team physician or athletic trainer.

_____ I will not return to play in a game or practice if I have received a blow to the head or body that results in concussion-related symptoms.

_____ Following concussion the brain needs time to heal. I understand that I am much more likely to have a repeat concussion if I return to play before symptoms resolve.

_____In rare cases, repeat concussions can cause permanent brain damage, and even death.

_____I have read and understand the signs and symptoms presented on the *Concussion Fact Sheet.*

_____   _____
Signature of Student-Athlete   Date

_____
Printed name of Student-Athlete

---

instances the clinician will have witnessed the concussive blow and has already established a mechanism of injury. However, if this is not possible, the athlete, teammates, coaches, or other personnel may provide beneficial information.[14] Obtaining a history through detailed questioning of the athlete about the injury will provide pertinent information relative to the injury. First, a level of consciousness can be established through dialog with the athlete. If the athlete is not alert enough to understand the questions or is passing in and out of consciousness, he or she should be transported to a medical facility for further evaluation. Second, the clinician can ascertain if the athlete is suffering from retrograde or anterograde amnesia. To establish the presence or absence of retrograde amnesia, injury history questions should start at the time of concussion and work backward. For example the clinician may ask: "do you remember getting hit?," "do you recall the play you were running?," "what team are we playing against?," and "what did you eat for breakfast or lunch?" Conversely, the assessment of anterograde amnesia should begin with questions surrounding events following the concussion, such as: "who was the first person you saw on the field?" or "who brought you to the sideline?" Providing the athlete with 3 unrelated words to recall at a later time (10–15-minute intervals) is also useful for assessing anterograde amnesia.

Box 2
Physician referral checklist

Day-of-Injury Referral

1. Loss of consciousness on the field

2. Amnesia lasting longer than 15 minutes

3. Deterioration of neurologic function[a]

4. Decreasing level of consciousness[a]

5. Decrease or irregularity in respirations[a]

6. Decrease or irregularity in pulse[a]

7. Increase in blood pressure

8. Unequal, dilated, or unreactive pupils[a]

9. Cranial-nerve deficits

10. Any signs or symptoms of associated injuries, spine or skull fracture, or bleeding[a]

11. Mental-status changes: lethargy, difficulty maintaining arousal, confusion, agitation[a]

12. Seizure activity[a]

13. Vomiting

14. Motor deficits subsequent to initial on-field assessment

15. Sensory deficits subsequent to initial on-field assessment

16. Balance deficits subsequent to initial on-field assessment

17. Cranial-nerve deficits subsequent to initial on-field assessment

18. Postconcussion symptoms that worsen

19. Additional postconcussion symptoms as compared with those on the field

20. Athlete is still symptomatic at the end of the game (especially at high school level)

Delayed Referral (After the Day of Injury)

1. Any of the findings in the day-of-injury referral category

2. Postconcussion symptoms worsen or do not improve over time

3. Increase in the number of postconcussion symptoms reported

4. Postconcussion symptoms begin to interfere with the athlete's daily activities (ie, sleep disturbances, cognitive difficulties)

[a] Requires the athlete be transported immediately to the nearest emergency department.
   Data from Guskiewicz KM, Bruce SL, Cantu RC, et al. National Athletic Trainers' Association Position Statement: management of sport-related concussion. J Athl Train 2004;29:280–97.

The sideline history evaluation should then follow with a series of questions addressing the presence or absence of a variety of concussion-related symptoms, and the severity of any symptoms. Several consensus groups have recommended the use of a graded symptom checklist for tracking the number, type, and severity of symptoms during serial assessments. The National Athletic Trainers' Association's Position Statement of Concussion Management recommends the use of a 27-item symptom checklist,[13] although several similar assessment tools are available.[15–17] These symptom scales use a Likert rating of severity that allows for an aggregate symptom severity score that can be used to track the severity over time. Tracking of the symptoms, as well as daily activities that might exacerbate symptoms, is strongly recommended (see example in **Fig. 1**). The presentation of symptoms will vary widely between concussed athletes, but some symptoms are reported to appear more often than others. For instance, headache has been reported in up to 83% of concussed athletes, while dizziness (65%) and confusion (57%) may also appear, but less frequently.[7,12,18,19] The clinician should recognize that some athletes removed from the field of play may report symptoms of dehydration (up to 2.5%) and not concussive injury.[20] Thus, the presence of symptoms in the absence of an insult to the head or torso may indicate dehydration rather than concussion. Regardless of

Concussion Graded Symptom Checklist (GSC) *(Grade symptoms 0-6)*					

Instructions: The GSC should be used not only for the initial evaluation but for each subsequent follow-up assessment until all signs and symptoms have cleared at rest and during physical exertion. In lieu of simply checking each symptom present, the ATC or physician can ask the athlete to grade or score the severity of the symptom 0-6, where 0=not present, 1=mild, 3=moderate, and 6=most severe.

Symptom	Date:	Date:	Date:	Date:	Date:
Blurred vision					
Dizziness					
Drowsiness					
Excess sleep					
Fatigue					
Feel "in a fog"					
Feel "slowed down"					
Headache					
Inappropriate emotions					
Irritability					
Memory problems					
Nausea					
Nervousness					
Poor balance/ coord.					
Poor concentration					
Ringing in ears					
Sadness					
Sensitivity to light					
Sensitivity to noise					
Sleep disturbance					
Daily Physical and Cognitive Activities:					

Fig. 1. The Graded Symptom Checklist (GCS).

which signs and symptoms appear, the endorsement of any symptom related to a concussion is sufficient to withhold an athlete from returning to play.[14]

Observation and palpation of the athlete can be completed throughout the injury evaluation process as the clinician interacts with the athlete. Attention should be paid to variance in the athlete's speech pattern from the norm, with difficulty finding or saying the correct words when responding to questions (ie, aphasia).[21] The clinician should also check equivalency of pupil size, their reaction to light, and the fluidity of eye movement in multiple directions (ie, nystagmus). Further, an evaluation of pulse and blood pressure should be completed to rule out a life-threatening condition. A high pulse pressure (ie, systolic minus diastolic >70 mm Hg) immediately following exercise is a common result of increased stroke volume,[22] but should be restored within 10 minutes. If the pulse pressure remains high and is combined with a pulse rate that is substantially lower than expected following physical exertion, the athlete may be suffering from increased intracranial pressure.[23] A clinical examination that reveals abnormalities in any of these areas suggests the injury is more significant than concussion, and warrants immediate transport and examination at a medical facility. The cervical spine and facial bones should also be palpated to rule out fractures or other trauma to these areas, which may be associated with high-acceleration impacts to the head.

Special tests used to evaluate for concussion on the sideline should consist of an evaluation of neuropsychological function, balance, and cranial nerve integrity. Although a variety of tests and questions have been recommended, traditional questions of orientation such as "where are you" and "what is your name?" have been found to be insensitive to the effects of concussion.[24,25] Alternatively, the Standardized Assessment of Concussion (SAC) was developed as a quick and reliable mental status examination for use on the sideline.[25] Different from more comprehensive pen-and-paper or computer-based neuropsychological assessments, the SAC does not require specific training in neuropsychology for the purposes of administration or interpretation.[26] These characteristics make it ideal for the practicing athletic trainer, who can administer the test in 6 to 8 minutes on the sideline.

The SAC consists of 5 sections that evaluate the areas of Orientation, Immediate Memory, Concentration, and Delayed Recall (**Fig. 2**). A brief screening has also been included to rule out gross neurologic deficiencies. Performance on each of the cognitive domains is summed for a total possible score of 30. The most accurate postmorbid assessment is completed when the postinjury score is compared with a preseason baseline assessment. Multiple versions of the SAC are available to reduce potential practice effects associated with multiple test administrations. Performance decrements of 1 point or more are consistent with impaired cognitive functioning following concussion. Specifically, when administered immediately following injury a 94% sensitivity and 76% specificity is obtained when a 1-point drop in test performance is used as a cutoff for concussion.[27] A follow-up investigation yielded similar sensitivity (80%) and specificity (91%) results when both concussed and control athletes were evaluated at similar time points following injury.[28]

One of the hallmark signs of concussion is a decreased ability to maintain balance. Concussed individuals will commonly show increased postural sway following injury, and the degree of sway will often increase when the eyes are closed, removing the visual referencing. Assessments of sway, such as the Romberg test, have been used,[29] but are limited by the subjective nature of postinjury interpretation. The Balance Error Scoring System (BESS) was developed as an objective postural control measure that can be implemented on the sideline.[30] The BESS test is conducted under 6 different stance conditions (**Fig. 3**): on a firm surface the athlete stands in

STANDARDIZED ASSESSMENT OF CONCUSSION - SAC | FORM C

NAME:_____

TEAM: _____ EXAMINER:_____

DATE OF EXAM: _____ TIME:_____

EXAM (Circle One): BLINE INJURY POST-PX/GAME
     DAY1   DAY2   DAY3   DAY5   DAY7   DAY90

INTRODUCTION:
I am going to ask you some questions.
Please listen carefully and give your best effort.

ORIENTATION

What Month is it?_____ 0   1
What's the Date today?_____ 0   1
What's the Day of Week?_____ 0   1
What Year is it?_____ 0   1
What Time is it right now? (within 1 hr.)_____ 0   1

Award 1 point for each correct answer.

ORIENTATION TOTAL SCORE [ ]

IMMEDIATE MEMORY

I am going to test your memory. I will read you a
list of words and when I am done, repeat back as
many words as you can remember, in any order.

LIST	TRIAL 1	TRIAL 2	TRIAL 3
BABY	0 1	0 1	0 1
MONKEY	0 1	0 1	0 1
PERFUME	0 1	0 1	0 1
SUNSET	0 1	0 1	0 1
IRON	0 1	0 1	0 1
TOTAL			

Trials 2 & 3: I am going to repeat that list again.
Repeat back as many words as you can remember
in any order, even if you said the word before.

Complete all 3 trials regardless of score on trial 1 & 2. 1 pt. for each
correct response. Total score equals sum across all 3 trials.

Do not inform the subject that delayed recall will be tested.

IMMEDIATE MEMORY TOTAL SCORE [ ]

EXERTIONAL MANEUVERS:

If subject is not displaying or reporting symptoms,
conduct the following maneuvers to create
conditions under which symptoms likely to be
elicited and detected. These measures need not be
conducted if a subject is already displaying or
reporting any symptoms. If not conducted, allow 2
minutes to keep time delay constant before testing
Delayed Recall. These methods should be
administered for baseline testing of normal subjects.

EXERTIONAL MANEUVERS	
5 Jumping Jacks	5 Push-Ups
5 Sit-ups	5 Knee Bends

© 1998 MCCREA, KELLY & RANDOLPH

NEUROLOGIC SCREENING

LOSS OF CONSCIOUSNESS/ WITNESSED UNRESPONSIVENESS	☐ No Length:	☐ Yes
POST-TRAUMATIC AMNESIA? Poor recall of events after injury	☐ No Length:	☐ Yes
RETROGRADE AMNESIA? Poor recall of events before injury	☐ No Length:	☐ Yes

	NORMAL	ABNORMAL
STRENGTH -		
Right Upper Extremity	☐	☐
Left Upper Extremity	☐	☐
Right Lower Extremity	☐	☐
Left Lower Extremity	☐	☐
SENSATION - examples: FINGER-TO-NOSE/ROMBERG	☐	☐
COORDINATION - examples: TANDEM WALK/ FINGER-NOSE-FINGER	☐	☐

CONCENTRATION

Digits Backward: I am going to read you a string of
numbers and when I am done, you repeat them
back to me backwards, in reverse order of how I
read them to you. For example, if I say 7-1-9, you
would say 9-1-7.
If correct, go to next string length. If incorrect, read trial 2. 1 pt.
possible for each string length. Stop after incorrect on both trials.

1-4-2	6-5-8	0 1
6-8-3-1	3-4-8-1	0 1
4-9-1-5-3	6-8-2-5-1	0 1
3-7-6-5-1-9	9-2-6-5-1-4	0 1

Months in Reverse Order: Now tell me the months
of the year in reverse order. Start with the last
month and go backward. So you'll say December,
November...Go ahead. 1 pt. for entire sequence correct

Dec-Nov-Oct-Sept-Aug-Jul-Jun-May-Apr-Mar-Feb-Jan   0   1

CONCENTRATION TOTAL SCORE [ ]

DELAYED RECALL

Do you remember that list of words I read a few
times earlier? Tell me as many words from the list
as you can remember in any order. Circle each word
correctly recalled. Total score equals number of words recalled.

BABY   MONKEY   PERFUME   SUNSET   IRON

DELAYED RECALL TOTAL SCORE [ ]

SAC SCORING SUMMARY

Exertional Maneuvers & Neurologic Screening are important for
examination, but not incorporated into SAC Total Score.

ORIENTATION	/ 5
IMMEDIATE MEMORY	/ 15
CONCENTRATION	/ 5
DELAYED RECALL	/ 5
SAC TOTAL SCORE	/30

Fig. 2. The Standardized Assessment of Concussion (SAC).

a double-leg stance, single-leg stance, and heel-to-toe tandem stance. The same 3 stances are repeated on a compliant foam surface such as an Airex balance pad (Alcan Airex AG, Switzerland). Each stance is evaluated for 20 seconds and the athlete places his or her hands on the hips with the eyes closed. During the trials the clinician counts the number of errors committed by the athlete (**Box 3**), with a higher number of errors representing suppressed balance. An increase of 3 errors or more over the baseline score has been suggested as a significant change indicating a balance

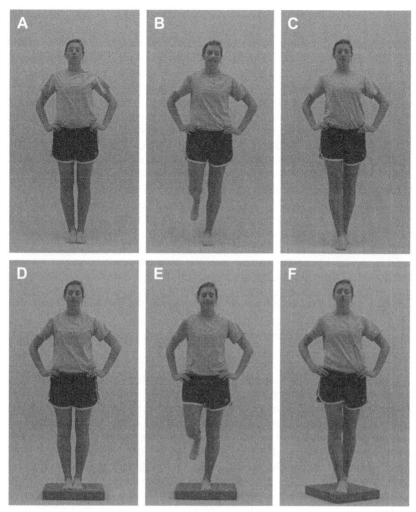

Fig. 3. Stances for the Balance Error Scoring System (BESS).

Box 3
Balance Error Scoring System countable errors
Errors
Hands lifted off the iliac crests
Opening eyes
Step, stumble, or fall
Moving the hip into more than 30° of flexion or extension
Lifting the forefoot or heel
Remaining out of the testing position for more than 5 seconds

impairment,[31] with a sensitivity to concussion reported at 34% and the specificity at 91%.[28]

Similar to the SAC assessment, an individualized approach to interpreting the post-injury BESS scores provides the clinician with the most accurate information. Thus, comparing the postconcussion assessment to the athlete's baseline assessment is recommended. To obtain the most accurate results, certain factors should be noted. For example, application of an external ankle support (eg, taping or bracing) has been shown to influence BESS scores.[32] Thus, when evaluating athletes on the sideline, it may be necessary to remove any ankle support that was not present at the time of baseline testing. Further, Wilkins and colleagues[33] noted a decrease in BESS performance when individuals were subjected to a 20-minute fatigue protocol. Athletes removed from a competition for an injury evaluation are likely experiencing some level of fatigue, necessitating some rest (13–20 minutes[34,35]) before testing.

Clinically meaningful deficits suggestive of neurologic impairment have been debated. However, as a general rule, an impact to the head with an accompanying increased symptom score, decreased SAC score (1 or more point[27]), or increased BESS score (3 or more points[31]) warrants removal from further participation. In the event SAC and BESS scores are normal in the postinjury evaluation and symptoms resolve within 20 minutes, the athlete should still be withheld from participation for the day.[14] Current practice guidelines set forth by the National Collegiate Athletic Association, National Football League, and National Hockey League all mandate that no player return to participation on the same day with a diagnosed concussion. Research supports this recommendation, as athletes have a higher likelihood of delayed symptom onset when returning to play on the same day in comparison with those withheld following the concussion.[7] Likewise, concussed athletes whose symptoms resolve within 25 minutes of injury have demonstrated impaired neuropsychological function 36 hours following the injury.[36]

Although complete disruption of one or more cranial nerves is rare in the sporting context, the clinician should also be cognizant that one or more of the cranial nerves may be affected as a result of the concussive blow. The assessment of many cranial nerves is imbedded throughout the concussion assessment (eg, cranial nerve II during the visual testing and cranial nerve VIII during the BESS test), but the integrity of the remaining nerves should be appraised as part of the sideline clinical assessment. A cranial-nerve assessment revealing functional decrements may also indicate a more severe injury causing increased intracranial pressure, and warrants a timely assessment at a medical facility.

Whereas the graded symptom checklist, SAC, and BESS have been discussed as options for special tests, other sideline assessment measures such as the Sideline Concussion Assessment Tool (ie, SCAT2)[37] have been proposed for a multifaceted sideline assessment tool to assess symptoms, cognitive function, and balance. The SCAT2 has shown promise, but to date it is limited by undefined psychometric properties and a lack of scientific studies validating its utility for concussion diagnosis and recovery.

Should the symptom reports, BESS scores, and SAC scores all appear normal, the clinician should continue with an evaluation of cervical ROM and strength testing. An examination of ROM for flexion, extension, and rotation in both directions should be conducted, both actively and passively. Similarly, manual muscle testing in the same directions should be performed. If limitations are noted in either ROM or muscle strength, the athlete should be withheld for further evaluation. Limitations in these areas may place the athlete at risk for further injury by restricting his or her ability to protect the head and anticipate for impacts from oncoming opponents.

Functional testing marks the final step in the sideline concussion assessment, but should not be confused with same-day return-to-play decision making. Rather, functional testing should only be completed if the athlete has performed at or above the baseline level of evaluation for symptoms, balance, and cognitive function, and if no other contraindications appear during the clinical examination. The goal of functional testing is to elicit symptoms that may present under the physical demands that the athlete might face after a return to play. A progressive approach to the physical activity should be taken, with the clinician asking if concussion-related symptoms have been elicited before moving to the next step. Simple tasks such as a Valsalva maneuver, push-ups, and sit-ups should be performed first; this may be followed by jogging and short sprints. In the final step the athlete should be able to complete a series of sport-specific activities at an intensity necessitated by the level of play. The clinician should ask the athlete at each progression to see if concussion-related symptoms have emerged. If the athlete indicates symptoms have resulted from the exertion, he or she should not be returned to participation or progressed to the next step in the graduated return-to-play progression. If no symptoms emerge and all other tests demonstrate normal findings, the athlete has likely not sustained a concussion and may be considered for a return to play.

SUMMARY

The evolution of sport-related concussion has brought technology and objective testing methods to the forefront of concussion management, not to mention an emphasis on concussion education, awareness, and prevention. Perhaps the greatest influence clinicians can have in preventing these injuries, or at least preventing catastrophic outcome, is to educate athletes, coaches, and parents about the dangers of playing while symptomatic following a concussion. Second only to this would be the implementation of a well-established concussion policy and emergency action plan. Contemporary methods of concussion assessment, involving the use of symptom checklists, neuropsychological testing, and postural stability testing, are indicated for any athlete suspected of having sustained a concussion, and research has shown the utility of these when incorporated into a systematic sideline assessment. Following a primary survey the clinician should garner an injury history, and observe and palpate the athlete for indications of more severe trauma. Special tests for mental status and postural control, along with reports of concussion-related symptoms, can provide the objective information that supports the clinical examination. Throughout the evaluation process the clinician should inquire about the development, presence, intensity, or return of concussion-related symptoms. In no instance should an athlete be returned to play if he or she reports any symptoms consistent with concussion, substantiating the dictum "when in doubt, sit them out."[38]

REFERENCES

1. Aubry M, Cantu R, Dvorak J, et al. Summary and agreement statement of the first International Conference on Concussion in Sport, Vienna 2001. Br J Sports Med 2002;36:6–10.
2. McCrory P, Johnston K, Meeuwisse W, et al. Summary and agreement statement of the second International Conference on Concussion in Sport, Prague 2004. Br J Sports Med 2005;39:196–204.
3. Hootman JM, Dick R, Agel J. Epidemiology of collegiate injuries for 15 sports: summary and recommendations for injury prevention initiatives. J Athl Train 2007;42(2):311–9.

4. Agel J, Dick R, Nelson B, et al. Descriptive epidemiology of collegiate women's ice hockey injuries: National Collegiate Athletic Association Injury Surveillance System, 2000-2001 through 2003-2004. J Athl Train 2007;42:249–54.
5. Broglio SP, Eckner JT, Surma T, et al. Post-concussion cognitive declines and symptomatology are not related to concussion biomechanics in high school football players. J Neurotrauma, in press.
6. Guskiewicz KM, Mihalik JP, Shankar V, et al. Measurement of head impacts in collegiate football players: relationship between head impact biomechanics and acute clinical outcome after concussion. Neurosurgery 2007;61:1244–52.
7. Guskiewicz KM, McCrea M, Marshall SW, et al. Cumulative effects associated with recurrent concussion in collegiate football players: the NCAA concussion study. JAMA 2003;290:2549–55.
8. Collins MW, Grindel SH, Lovell MR, et al. Relationship between concussion and neuropsychological performance in college football players. JAMA 1999;282:964–70.
9. Field M, Collins MW, Lovell MR, et al. Does age play a role in recovery from sports-related concussion? A comparison of high school and collegiate athletes. J Pediatr 2003;142:546–53.
10. Grindel SH, Lovell MR, Collins MW. The assessment of sport-related concussion: the evidence behind neuropsychological testing and management. Clin J Sport Med 2001;11:134–43.
11. McCrea M, Hammeke T, Olsen G, et al. Unreported concussion in high school football players: implications for prevention. Clin J Sport Med 2004;14:13–7.
12. Delaney JS, Lacroix VJ, Leclerc S, et al. Concussions among university football and soccer players. Clin J Sport Med 2002;12:331–8.
13. Guskiewicz KM, Bruce SL, Cantu RC, et al. National Athletic Trainers' Association Position Statement: management of sport-related concussion. J Athl Train 2004; 29:280–97.
14. Broglio SP, Guskiewicz KM. Concussion in sport: the sideline assessment. Sports Health: A Multidisciplinary Approach 2009;1:361–9.
15. Piland SG, Motl RW, Ferrara MS, et al. Evidence for the factorial and construct validity of a self-report concussion symptoms scale. J Athl Train 2003;38:104–12.
16. Lovell MR, Collins MW. Neuropsychological assessment of the college football player. J Head Trauma Rehabil 1998;13:9–26.
17. Potter S, Leigh E, Wade D, et al. The Rivermead Post Concussion Symptoms Questionnaire: a confirmatory factor analysis. J Neurol 2006;253:1603–14.
18. McCrory PR, Ariens M, Berkovic SF. The nature and duration of acute concussive symptoms in Australian football. Clin J Sport Med 2000;10:235–8.
19. Guskiewicz K, Weaver NL, Padua DA, et al. Epidemiology of concussion in collegiate and high school football players. Am J Sports Med 2000;28:643–50.
20. Patel AV, Mihalik JP, Notebaert AJ, et al. Neuropsychological performance, postural stability, and symptoms after dehydration. J Athl Train 2007;42:66–75.
21. Ropper AH, Gorson KC. Clinical practice: concussion. N Engl J Med 2007;356: 166–72.
22. Dart AM, Kingwell BA. Pulse pressure—a review of mechanisms and clinical relevance. J Am Coll Cardiol 2001;37:975–84.
23. Sanders MJ, McKenna K. Head and facial trauma. Mosby's paramedic textbook. 2nd edition. St. Louis (MO): Mosby; 2001. p. 624–51.
24. Maddocks DL, Dicker GD, Saling MM. The assessment of orientation following concussion in athletes. Clin J Sport Med 1995;5:32–5.
25. McCrea M, Kelly JP, Kluge J, et al. Standardized assessment of concussion in football players. Neurology 1997;48:586–8.

26. McCrea M. Standardized mental status assessment of sports concussion. Clin J Sport Med 2001;11:176–81.
27. Barr WB, McCrea M. Sensitivity and specificity of standardized neurocognitive testing immediately following sports concussion. J Int Neuropsychol Soc 2001; 7:693–702.
28. McCrea M, Barr WB, Guskiewicz KM, et al. Standard regression-based methods for measuring recovery after sport-related concussion. J Int Neuropsychol Soc 2005;11:58–69.
29. Romberg MH. A manual of the nervous disease of man. London: Sydenham Society; 1853.
30. Riemann BL, Guskiewicz KM, Shields EW. Relationship between clinical and forceplate measures of postural stability. J Sport Rehab 1999;8:71–82.
31. Valovich McLeod TC, Barr WB, McCrea M, et al. Psychometric and measurement properties of concussion assessment tools in youth sports. J Athl Train 2006;41: 399–408.
32. Broglio SP, Monk A, Sopiarz K, et al. The influence of ankle support on postural control. J Sci Med Sport 2009;12:388–92.
33. Wilkins JC, Valovich TC, Perrin DH, et al. Performance on the Balance Error Scoring System decreases after fatigue. J Athl Train 2004;39:156–61.
34. Susco TM, Valovich McLeod TC, Gansneder BM, et al. Balance recovers within 20 minutes after exertion as measured by the Balance Error Scoring System. J Athl Train 2004;39:241–6.
35. Fox ZG, Mihalik JP, Blackburn JT, et al. Return of postural control to baseline after anaerobic and aerobic exercise protocols. J Athl Train 2008;43:456–63.
36. Lovell MR, Collins MW, Iverson GL, et al. Grade 1 or "ding" concussions in high school athletes. Am J Sports Med 2004;32:47–54.
37. McCrory P, Meeuwisse W, Johnston K, et al. Consensus Statement on Concussion in Sport, 3rd International Conference on Concussion in Sport Held in Zurich, November 2008. Br J Sports Med 2009;43:i76–90.
38. Cantu RC. Athletic concussion: current understanding as of 2007. Neurosurgery 2007;60:963–4.

Return-to-Play Decisions

Scott R. Laker, MD

KEYWORDS

• Sport • Concussion • Brain • Post-concussion syndrome

Sports concussions are mild traumatic brain injuries, and all brain injuries are serious. The most recent Concussion in Sport consensus statement states "Concussion is defined as a complex pathophysiologic process affecting the brain, induced by traumatic biomechanical forces." Concussions occur as a result of forces directed to the head or neck, or from impulsive forces transmitted from the body to the head. They result in the rapid onset and spontaneous recovery of short-lived impairment of neurologic function.[1] Concussions represent a functional disturbance and not a structural one, and do not result in abnormalities on standard structural imaging. A concussion results in a graded set of clinical symptoms that do not have to result in loss of consciousness (LOC). These symptoms resolve in a stepwise fashion in most cases. A small minority of cases result in prolonged symptoms referred to as postconcussion syndrome (PCS).[1]

The Centers for Disease Control (CDC) estimates between 1.6 and 3.8 million sports and recreation concussions occur each year, and that approximately 135,000 sports concussions are seen in emergency departments annually.[2–4] This estimate has increased greatly since the CDC's previous estimate of 300,000 sports and recreation concussions in 1997.[5] It is likely that this is because of an increased awareness of the injury rather than an intrinsic change in the rate of concussion.

The improved medical understanding of concussion, combined with an increased awareness in the nonmedical press, has pushed concussion management to the forefront of sideline and clinical sports medicine. Legislation exists in several states that addresses same-day return to play (RTP) and medical clearance before full RTP. As the number of concussion cases presenting in clinics has increased, the challenge of making evidence-based RTP decisions has become apparent.

Yard and Comstock[6] report that high school athletes returned to sport prematurely in 40.5% of cases based on data from the American Academy of Neurology (AAN), and in 15% of cases using the 2005 Prague Consensus Statement guidelines. Yard and Comstock[6] also report that 15.8% of football players suffering a concussion with

The author has nothing to disclose.
Department of Physical Medicine and Rehabilitation, University of Colorado, Mail Stop F493, 12631 East 17th Avenue, Room 2513, Aurora, CO 80045, USA
E-mail address: scott.laker@ucdenver.edu

Phys Med Rehabil Clin N Am 22 (2011) 619–634
doi:10.1016/j.pmr.2011.08.004
1047-9651/11/$ – see front matter © 2011 Published by Elsevier Inc.

LOC returned to play on the same day as their injury. The increased media attention, law changes, and overall awareness of the seriousness of the condition suggest that compliance will improve, although this remains to be seen. This article discusses a comprehensive approach to RTP in sports concussion, including managing athletes returning after prolonged PCS, multiple concussions, and intracranial hematomas and craniotomy.

PATHOPHYSIOLOGY AND RTP

An understanding of the pathophysiology of concussion and the cellular dysfunction that occurs guides the approach to an athlete's eventual RTP. Current understanding of the pathophysiology of concussion supports the neurometabolic cascade theory, which has been well described elsewhere[7,8] (please see the article by Schrey and colleagues elsewhere in this issue for details). It theorizes that concussions result in microscopic cellular damage and disruption of the normal equilibrium of the cellular membrane. This disruption and axonal stretch causes a cellular depolarization and release of excitatory amino acids and disrupts the ionic balance in the cell. The Na^+/K^+ ATP-dependent pump initiates to regain the cell's normal ionic balance. This energy-dependent, glycolytic pathway eventually leads to lactate accumulation. Ca^{2+} rushes into the mitochondria and inhibits oxidative processes. These intracellular processes lead to, and are accompanied by, secondary damage to the axonal substructure.[7]

There is an initial hyperglycolysis that occurs immediately after the injury and may last up to 30 minutes. This hyperglycolysis quickly transforms into a glucose hypometabolism that may last for days. In more severe brain injury, there is well-described impaired cerebral blood flow that limits the ability of the cells to acquire more glucose.[7,9–11] The increase in the brain's intracellular demands, combined with a supply-side limitation in glucose, is theorized to lead to the clinical features of concussion. This supply-and-demand mismatch may explain the common complaint that mental and physical exertion exacerbate or uncover symptoms in patients who are asymptomatic at rest.

EPIDEMIOLOGY AND RTP

Concussion epidemiology data have been reported for multiple sports, age groups, and competition levels[12–17] (see the article by Jinguji and colleagues elsewhere in this issue for further details). The highest overall number of concussions occur in men's football and in women's ice hockey. Recent data indicate the overall rate of concussion in high school to be 0.23 per 1000 athlete exposures.[18] The collegiate rate is higher at 0.43 per 1000 athlete exposures.[12]

The terms simple and complex are based on duration of symptoms, and the Zurich consensus statement states that these terms have limited usefulness.[19] There is no mechanism to prospectively predict which athletes will have prolonged recoveries, making this distinction of limited value. Discussing recovery timeframes with athletes is reasonable, because 80% to 90% of youth athletes improve within 7 to 10 days.[19] However, all concussions are not equal, and a 3-month recovery is different than a 3-day recovery. It is not yet possible to factor these differences into practical management, and there is a limited amount of information available specifically for recovery from more severe concussions.[20]

Athletes with a history of previous concussion are more likely to have repeat concussions than their nonconcussed counterparts.[21] Athletes with 3 or more concussions are more than 3 times as likely to suffer a concussion than their nonconcussed counterparts.[21] Athletes with a history of more than 3 previous concussions have a more severe sideline presentation, including LOC, anterograde amnesia, confusion, and overall number of symptoms.[22] In a large study of nearly 17,000 high school and collegiate athletes, the rate of repeat concussion within the same season is reported to be 3.8%, and 79.2% of these athletes with second concussions occurred within 7 days of the first concussion.[17] These are compelling data to suggest that even a youth athlete in whom symptoms resolve rapidly should not RTP within 7 days of the initial concussion, although this is not a defined standard of care. There is no current way to predict which athletes are at risk for the repeat first-week concussions.

Modifying factors associated with prolonged PCS include history of depression, mental health disorders, migraine, headache disorder, attention deficit and hyperactivity disorder, learning disability, and sleep disorders.[23–25] **Table 1** summarizes the full spectrum of modifying factors associated with PCS.[19] These modifying factors should be identified in athletes presenting with concussion, but there is no clear way of using them in RTP decisions.

SAME-DAY RETURN-TO-PLAY

There is consensus that no youth athlete with a concussion should return to play on the same day as the initial injury.[19] Multiple national and international organizations have position statements or clinical papers that support this position, including the National Athletic Trainer's Association and American Academy of Pediatrics.[26] The AAN has issued a practice reference sheet and is preparing an updated guideline for late 2011.[27] The National Collegiate Activities Association (NCAA) has mandated that schools have concussion management plans and have precluded same-day

Table 1 Modifying factors in concussion	
Factors	**Modifiers**
Symptoms	Number
	Duration (>10 d)
	Severity
Signs	Prolonged LOC, amnesia
Sequelae	Convulsions
Temporal	Frequency
	Timing
	Recency
Threshold	Repeated concussions with less impact
	Slower recovery
Age	Children and adolescents
Comorbidity	Migraine, depression, or other mental health disorders, ADHD, LD, sleep disorders
Medications	Psychoactive drugs, anticoagulants
Behavior	Dangerous style of play
Sport	High-risk activity, contact and collision sport, high sporting level

Abbreviations: ADHD, attention deficit hyperactivity disorder; LD, learning disability.

From McCrory P, Meeuwisse W, Johnston K, et al. Consensus statement on Concussion in Sport: the 3rd International Conference on Concussion in Sport held in Zurich, November 2008. Br J Sports Med 2009;43(Suppl 1):i79.

RTP, stating in their most recent Sports Medicine Handbook that "Student-athletes diagnosed with a concussion shall not return to activity for the remainder of that day. Medical clearance shall be determined by the team physician or his or her designee according to the concussion management plan."[28]

The current Concussion in Sport consensus statement states that same-day RTP can be considered in select, adult populations in which there is sideline access to experienced physicians, neuropsychologists, neuroimaging, and sideline access to neurocognitive assessment. The National Football League has stated that "Once removed for the duration of a practice or game, the player should not be considered for return-to-football activities until he is fully asymptomatic, both at rest and after exertion, has a normal neurologic examination, normal neuropsychological testing, and has been cleared to return by both his team physician(s) and the independent neurologic consultant."[29] The principles of asymptomatic RTP are still in effect in this select scenario, and full symptom and cognitive recovery must take place before same-day RTP may be considered. In clinical practice, this scenario is limited to professional sports and an adult population.

SECOND-IMPACT SYNDROME

The most devastating complication in sports concussion is second-impact syndrome (SIS). This is a clinical syndrome in which an athlete suffers a concussion and returns to play before the symptoms have resolved. A second traumatic insult occurs, usually involving a smaller impact, and a rapid deterioration in neurologic status is observed, leading to death within minutes from primary cerebral swelling and cerebellar herniation. Imaging and autopsy classically reveal no intracranial bleeding. These clinical factors define SIS.[30] There are increasing numbers of cases that involve a small amount of intracranial bleeding in the presence of massive cerebral swelling. These small hematomas do not account for the severity of the clinical outcomes. Most of the reported cases have been in athletes less than 18 years old, although there are cases of older athletes within the literature.[31,32]

The rapidity of neurologic decline and the extreme nature of the brain swelling suggest a problem with the brain's ability to autoregulate, which corresponds with the current understanding of concussion pathophysiology. In a rat mild traumatic brain injury (mTBI) model, all animals received a first mTBI and then a second was induced at intervals of 1, 3, or 7 days after the first. No rat deaths were reported in the control group (single mTBI), whereas 10% of rats died in the double-impact group. In addition, the cellular and mitochondrial changes seen were more significant than those with a single injury.[10] Rat model data suggest that the glucose metabolism may be altered up to 10 days after the initial injury and Ca^{2+} derangements up to 4 days after single injury, and concerns exist that these time periods may be longer in humans.[7] These animal model findings help support the concept of no same-day RTP, although further research is necessary to help identify the application of this theory in humans.

Probable or definite SIS is exceedingly rare and no true incidence is known. Arguments have been made that RTP protocols are based largely on fear of SIS.[33] The cases of SIS are devastating to families and communities and are highly publicized in the medical and lay press. It is the most severe outcome of concussion and cannot be ignored. There is no evidence to suggest that athletes with a history of multiple concussions have a greater likelihood of SIS, although the small number of reported SIS cases makes this a tentative statement. Nonetheless, there are many more common consequences of premature RTP and early exertion, like prolongation of symptoms and poor neurocognitive performance.[34,35]

CURRENT RTP PROTOCOL

No athlete should RTP while still suffering from symptoms. This recommendation is consistent throughout the literature. The Zurich consensus statement outlines a framework from which to approach an athlete who has recovered from the symptoms of a concussion and is ready to begin working toward a return to competition (**Table 2**).[1] Each stage should take 24 hours before advancing to the next stage. If athletes experiences a return of their symptoms, they should stop advancing and return to the previous stage. They should remain at the previous stage for 24 hours before attempting the next stage in the RTP protocol. This protocol takes approximately 1 week to complete, assuming that the athlete remains asymptomatic. However, this protocol may take weeks or months to complete depending on the athlete's response to the increasing exertion.

There is some discussion in the Zurich consensus statement that the elite, adult athlete may RTP more rapidly than the nonelite athlete.[1] This concept was recently echoed by Putukian and colleagues.[36] This idea is based more on access to experienced medical professionals than on a difference in pathology or recovery. For example, a professional or NCAA athlete may have immediate, daily access to a trainer, neuropsychologist, physician, and concussion specialist. This access combined with the high experience level of the medical team may translate into faster RTP. However, this concept of rapid RTP is controversial and currently has no level I evidence to support it. This expedited model of RTP currently has no role for the nonelite, youth athlete.

Athletes who have had prolonged postconcussion syndrome may take longer to progress through these stages, although this may be because of underlying deconditioning from lack of activity rather than a difference in neurocognitive recovery. The provider should be aware of these issues to prevent other injuries from overzealous

Table 2 RTP progression		
Rehabilitation Stage	**Functional Exercise at Each Stage of Rehabilitation**	**Objective of Each Stage**
1. No activity	Complete physical and cognitive rest	Recovery
2. Light aerobic exercise	Walking, swimming, or stationary cycling keeping intensity <70% MPHR. No resistance training	Increase HR
3. Sport-specific exercise	Skating drills in ice hockey, running drills in soccer. No head-impact activities	Add movement
4. Noncontact training drills	Progression to more complex training drills (eg, passing drills in football and ice hockey). May start progressive resistance training	Exercise, coordination, cognitive load
5. Full-contact practice	Following medical clearance, participate in normal training activities	Restore confidence, assessment of functional skills by coaching staff
6. RTP	Normal game play	

Abbreviations: HR, heart rate; MPHR, maximum predicted heart rate.
From McCrory P, Meeuwisse W, Johnston K, et al. Consensus statement on Concussion in Sport: the 3rd International Conference on Concussion in Sport held in Zurich, November 2008. Br J Sports Med 2009;43(Suppl 1):i79.

athletes returning to full competition before they are physically prepared. Athletes who have months of symptoms should start a conditioning and training program similar to athletes with musculoskeletal injuries that require significant loss of participation time.

NEUROPSYCHOLOGICAL DATA AND RTP

Neuropsychological (NP) testing abnormalities are well described in the literature, and the National Academy of Neuropsychology has issued a position paper on the use in concussed athletes.[37-39] Because the treatment protocols have changed to restrict any symptomatic athlete from returning, the role of NP testing is still debated. Several studies have found that NP abnormalities resolve in parallel with symptom resolution. If this were true in every case of concussion, the usefulness of NP testing might be called into question. There are several other studies that indicate that NP testing may resolve more slowly than symptoms.[40-42] This would suggest that NP testing offers another degree of assurance that an athlete has fully recovered and can begin an RTP program. Athletes who undergo NP testing tend to RTP more slowly than their nontested counterparts.[43]

NP testing results are not a substitute for clinical judgment and a return to baseline on NP testing is only 1 component of RTP decision making. NP testing becomes increasingly useful as the duration of symptoms expands to track neurocognitive improvement. The neuropsychologist also has the ability to screen for comorbid and preexisting conditions like anxiety, depression, undiagnosed learning disability, and others that may affect clinical decision making and potential interventions. In student athletes, NP testing may help guide school accommodations and help more objectively document cognitive dysfunction. Student athletes who have severely prolonged PCS should have clear medical and NP documentation of their condition as they move forward to prevent problems during the high school or college admissions process.

PSYCHOLOGICAL CONSIDERATIONS

As acute symptoms move into chronic PCS, the interplay of nonorganic, social, and psychological factors becomes increasingly important. Jacobson discusses the issues of physiogenesis and psychogenesis as they relate to PCS.[44] Premorbid mental and physical health status were more predictive of persistent PCS than head injury severity (as defined by LOC and posttraumatic amnesia) in a study of adults with mild TBI.[45] PCS has also been described as an environmental stress combined with an individual predisposition to the injury or syndrome.[46] Preconcussion depressive symptoms may alter baseline neuropsychological testing.[47] Interventions to help an athlete address these issues include consulting a sports psychologist, biofeedback, visualization exercises, support groups, and reintegration into social groups.

Recovery from sports injuries are classically believed to follow the stages of grief hypothesized by Kübler-Ross,[48] including denial, anger, bargaining, depression, and acceptance.[48] The grief model in athletes tends not to involve the denial stage prominently.[49] Wiese-bjornstal and colleagues[50] created a model to identify the factors affecting an athlete with a sports injury. A comparison study between athletes with anterior cruciate ligament (ACL) injuries and concussion found that both groups had increased depression scores. The ACL group had more significant and longer-lasting changes. The concussed group had depression scores that lasted approximately 1 week and a more severe total mood disturbance at day 4.[51] This finding may reflect that the depression experience by the acutely concussed athlete is a direct result of the concussion, rather than a situational depression. There is significant over-lap between the symptoms of depression and those of PCS as shown by Iverson[52] who found that almost 50% of depressed patients without current concussion endorsed symptoms at a clinically significant level for PCS as defined by the DSM-IV. Alternative diagnoses must be ruled out to decrease attribution error (ie, all subse-quent symptoms attributed to the concussion). To some extent, stigma still surrounds anxiety and depression and it may be more socially acceptable for an athlete and/or their families to attribute symptoms to a sports injury rather than to an underlying psychiatric condition.

In the professional athlete, these issues include the concern of loss of livelihood. Media exposure of the injury adds to the pressure on both the athlete and the treating physician to return an athlete as quickly as possible. As with all team physicians, the primary responsibility is to athletes and their health.

Athletes returning to play face several issues not directly related to their concussion. These issues commonly include fear of repeat concussion, concern for future disability, and performance anxiety. Many athletes suffer from the loss of a sense of invincibility and decrease in overall health during the recovery from concussion. Isola-tion and lack of social support during the removal from practice and play is a common stressor for concussed athletes. There is increasing awareness about the role of anxiety and depression as direct sequelae of concussion. Concern exists that the treatment of concussion (prolonged rest) may lead to depressed mood, fatigue, and irritability. Aerobic, anaerobic, and resistance exercise have beneficial mood effects and alter the brain's neurochemistry. The removal of exercise combined with the cascade of neurometabolic changes may exacerbate these mood disturbances. Athletes in whom low-grade symptoms linger for several weeks may consider a trial of gentle aerobic exercise in efforts to remove these iatrogenic causes for prolonged PCS. A recent preliminary safety study on concussed patients with more than 6 weeks of symptoms using an incremental treadmill protocol showed that the athletes were able to exercise at near age-predicted heart rate maximum without symptom exacer-bation. The patients had symptom improvement that corresponded with their peak heart rate.[53] This study is promising but small (n = 12). Larger numbers of patients and reproducible results are needed before expanding this to nonexperimental popu-lations. Athletes should not be returned to a contact situation until they are fully asymptomatic.

It is wise to discuss these issues proactively with an athlete as they are beginning their RTP protocols and intervening early to limit any undue psychological distress that an athlete may encounter.

PERSISTING HEADACHE AND RTP

The most common symptom after concussion and in PCS is headache (please see the article by Blume and colleagues elsewhere in this issue for further details). Given the functional problems caused by headache, increasing numbers of concussed athletes are started on prescription medications. As these athletes improve and become asymptomatic, the question arises as to how to return medicated athletes to play (ie, are they asymptomatic simply because of the medication?). To the author's knowl-edge, no literature exists to guide this decision. Several of the medications used for headache in this population may require several days to weeks to taper. It is this author's recommendation to allow athletes with PCS who are started on medications beyond simple over-the-counter medications to remain asymptomatic for at least 1 month before progressing aerobic exercise. If symptoms return, it is up to the treating physician to use clinical judgment to determine whether the symptoms are caused by incomplete resolution of symptoms, deconditioning, or a newly diagnosed posttraumatic headache disorder. Consultation with a headache specialist can help guide these decisions.

LONG-TERM SEQUELAE

A significant concern for athletes with multiple concussions is the possibility for long-term deficits. Although most athletes with concussion have no lasting deficits, there are increasing reports of long-term effects of concussion in certain athletes. These effects may include neuropsychiatric, somatic, and cognitive impairment.[21,54] Chronic traumatic encephalopathy (CTE) has become an increasingly recognized phenomenon. It is likely that CTE was the cause of dementia pugilistica and punch-drunk syndromes. Omalu and colleagues[55–58] have published several case reports with confirmed CTE. Cantu and colleagues[59] at the Sports Legacy Institute have published widely on this as well.[60] Factors common to cases with confirmed CTE include professional sporting career, a history of multiple subconcussive head impacts, and symptomatic concussions.

SEASON TERMINATION AND RETIREMENT CONSIDERATIONS

Several published guidelines for the termination of a season exist, although they are based on concussion grading scales that are no longer the standard of care (**Table 3**).[61–63] There are also published reviews that have addressed this topic.[64,65] As previously discussed, concussion management is individualized and algorithmic approaches to retirement should be avoided. Nevertheless, an understanding of the historical framework may help the clinician to formulate management plans for their multiply concussed athletes. The previously published guidelines are based heavily on LOC, which has limited correlation with symptom duration or severity. The AAN is issuing new guidelines later in 2011 and no longer uses concussion grades.[66]

Decisions regarding RTP in athletes with multiple concussions are based on multiple factors. Each subsequent concussion makes an athlete statistically more likely to sustain a further concussion, and concerns exist regarding the potential for progressively long symptom duration after multiple concussions.[21,67,68] There is no defined number of concussions that is too many. Many of the data available on epidemiology indicate that previous history of concussion increases the risk for future injury. These factors should be discussed at length with the patient. The 3-strikes-and-out paradigm is still a commonly held approach toward concussion management. As with most RTP concepts, this is based on expert opinion and a paucity of literature. There is no evidence to suggest that athletes with more than 3 concussions are at increased risk for PCS.[69] There is an absence of evidence regarding athletes with prolonged symptoms after a first concussion to suggest that they are at risk of similar clinical trajectories for subsequent concussions.

Zemper[68] prospectively found that high school and college athletes with a history of self-reported concussion had a nearly sixfold relative risk of future concussions in the following 2 seasons. This study did not analyze for a history of multiple concussions, so dose-response information is unknown. Guskiewicz and colleagues[21] reported that athletes with history of 3 previous concussions were 3 times more likely to have a subsequent concussion. Athletes with 3 or more concussions have more severe on-field presentations after subsequent concussions.[22] Athletes with 3 or more concussions have longer postconcussion symptom duration than athletes without

Table 3
Previous recommendations regarding multiple concussions

	Grade	First Concussion	Second Concussion	Third Concussion
Cantu[63] (2001 revised)	Grade 1 (mild)	May RTP if asymptomatic for 1 wk	May return to play in 2 wk, if asymptomatic for 1 wk	Terminate season, return if asymptomatic next season
	Grade 2 (moderate)	May return to play if asymptomatic for 1 wk	Minimum 1 mo, may return to play if asymptomatic for 1 wk. Consider terminating season	Terminate season, return if asymptomatic next season
	Grade 3 (severe)	Minimum of 1 mo, may return to play if asymptomatic for 1 wk	Terminate season, return if asymptomatic next season	
AAN[81]	Grade 1: no LOC, confusion lasting <15 min	RTP in 15 min if asymptomatic	RTP in 1 wk if asymptomatic. Remove from play if 2 concussions in same day	RTP in 1 wk if asymptomatic
	Grade 2: no LOC, confusion lasting longer than 15 min	RTP when asymptomatic for 1 wk	RTP in 2 wk if asymptomatic	RTP in 2 wk if asymptomatic
	Grade 3: any LOC	RTP when asymptomatic for 1 wk	RTP after 1 mo	RTP after 1 mo or longer, at provider's discretion
Colorado[82]	Grade 1: no LOC, confusion, or amnesia	RTP in 20 min if asymptomatic	RTP if asymptomatic for 1 wk	Terminate season. RTP next season if asymptomatic
	Grade 2: no LOC, confusion, amnesia	RTP after a minimum of 1 wk with no symptoms	RTP after a minimum of 1 mo with no symptoms for 1 wk	Terminate season. RTP next season if asymptomatic
	Grade 3: any duration of LOC	RTP after a minimum of 2 wk with no symptoms	Terminate season. RTP next season if asymptomatic	Terminate season. RTP next season if asymptomatic

Please note that grades of concussions are no longer used for decision making for individual players. This table is presented for historical perspective.

concussion history. Thirty percent of multiply concussed athletes had more than 7 days of symptoms compared with 14.6% of athletes with no history of concussion.[21]

Collins and colleagues[70] found that athletes with ≥ 2 concussions had more deficit-son the Trailmaking Test and the Symbol Digit Modalities Test when compared to athletes with 1 concussion and athletes with no history of concussion. De Beaumont and colleagues[71] found that retired university-level athletes had deficits on cognitive and motor testing decades after their last reported concussion. This study also revealed abnormalities on neuropsychological and electrophysiologic measures of memory.[71] Covassin and colleagues[72] found a dose-response relationship on ImPACT testing in male and female athletes with more than 2 previous self-reported concussions. Kuehl and colleagues[73] found that athletes with more than 3 concussions scored lower on the bodily pain, vitality, and social functioning sections of the Short Form 36 than did their nonconcussed counterparts.

There are several circumstances in which retirement should be recommended to an athlete. All of the retirement recommendations can be considered level IV evidence and are based largely on expert opinion. Absolute contraindications to return to competition include ongoing symptoms, abnormal neurologic examination, NP testing that has not returned to baseline, or imaging that indicates that the athlete is at increased risk for repeat injury.[64] Given that NP testing is used to determine appropriateness of retirement, it is reasonable to obtain high-quality NP baseline data in athletes with a history of multiple or severe concussions in whom retirement is a potential outcome, as a reference for subsequent RTP decisions. These absolute contraindications are rare but should not be missed. Relative contraindications include symptoms that last months and not days, or decreased injury threshold (concussions that arise from minimal contact).[64]

Cantu[74] proposed that retirement should be considered in the presence of more than 3 concussions combined with increasing recovery times (especially >3 months) and decreasing injury threshold forces. Of similar concern is the athlete who displays several months of symptoms after the first concussion. This scenario has not been well addressed in the literature and no evidence-based conclusions can be made. The literature is beginning to support the widely held clinical assumption that multiple concussions create the potential for long-term sequelae, including cognitive dysfunction, increased symptom report, depression, and, potentially, CTE.[21,59,60,75–77] These concerns should be part of the informed consent as an athlete considers RTP after multiple concussions.

INTRACRANIAL LESIONS AND RTP

Intracranial bleeding is a serious and potentially life-threatening injury. Improved medical care and access to trauma centers ensures that athletes who suffer intracranial hematomas are more likely to survive and may recover without significant disability. In these athletes, the question remains as to when, whether, and how to return them to contact sports.

There is no level I evidence to guide these decisions. The case reports and editorial by Davis and colleagues[78] is an excellent discussion of the considerations for RTP in an athlete with an intracranial bleed. Before consideration of RTP, an extradural hematoma must be fully resolved and the fracture fully healed. In subdural hematomas, the hematoma must be resolved, the brain reexpanded to fill the subdural space, and there must be no residual hygroma. A thorough workup for risk factors must be negative, to include coagulopathy and risk-producing brain abnormalities.[78] It is reasonable to add that a return to normal NP baseline should also be a prerequisite for RTP consideration. The timeframes mentioned are based largely on healing times for the fracture and the reabsorption times of the hematoma, and are estimated to be 1 year.

There is also no level I evidence to guide a physician considering RTP in athletes after craniotomy. There have been few reports on return to collision or contact sport after craniotomy and many of them are in the lay press. There have been cases of a professional hockey player, professional boxers, an amateur soccer player, and a professional footballer returning to their sport after craniotomy.[79] Expert opinion is that RTP can be considered after complete bony union is documented and neurologic, radiological, and neuropsychological evidence of recovery is documented. RTP may depend on to which sport the athlete is returning. For example, Davis and colleagues[78] did not agree on whether to return a boxer to competition after complete resolution after craniotomy, whereas a soccer player would be returned provided a well-fitted helmet be worn during competition. Rigid bone flap fixation methods are perhaps more stable and may allow athletes to return more quickly, although this has not been studied.

In the author's experience, the decision to return an athlete to competition after an intracranial bleed or craniotomy is done no earlier than 1 year after the injury and is based on the input of a team consisting of a neurosurgeon, neuroradiologist, neuropsychologist, and sports medicine physician.

MEDIOCOLEGAL ASPECTS OF RTP

The Health Information Privacy and Portability Act (HIPPA) defines the framework for communication of patient information. The team physician and the consulting physician are both bound by HIPPA. It is recommended that providers obtain written consent regarding disclosure of patient information as it relates to a concussed athlete. It is common for providers caring for concussed athletes to be asked to discuss the case with trainers, coaches, teachers, guidance counselors, and other physicians. It must be clearly documented that consent to release medical information has been granted before these discussions. Consider having a formal policy based on state law and your institution's legal counsel. Pearsall and colleagues[80] review this and similar issues.

Multiple states now require written clearance before an athlete may return to competition after an acute concussion. In states with legislation regarding written RTP clearance, an athlete may not return without clearance. The difficulty arises in cases in which the team physician or coach is aware that a physician has cleared an athlete and another has recommended no RTP. The team physician should adhere to the standards of care discussed within this article and elsewhere to guide decisions on RTP and obtain specialist consultation in complicated cases. Even in the presence of written physician clearance, if a coach or team physician has concerns that the athlete is still symptomatic, the athlete should be removed from play until it is clear that the athlete is safe to return.

The medicolegal aspects of RTP in multiply concussed athletes or athletes with prolonged PCS are less clear. The main questions in disputed cases are whether an athlete can decide to return to competition despite a medical recommendation to retire or terminate a season, and whether an athlete can sign a liability waiver that removes the risk of future litigation. Both scenarios are fraught with potential for litigation. An athlete returning to sport in a disputed case relies on the team physician and the institution governing that athletic endeavor, combined with expert medical opinion and legal advice.

DISCUSSION

Concussion management needs to expand its literature base to help guide clinical decisions. Current RTP recommendations are based on expert opinion using the available epidemiologic data, pathophysiology theories, NP testing literature, and retrospective clinical studies. The strongest recommendation is that no athlete should RTP while symptomatic. Most youth athletes improve within 7 to 10 days and are unlikely to require specific medical interventions beyond education on acute concussion management and avoidance of repeat injury. RTP should be a medically supervised, stepwise plan that occurs in the course of a week (see **Table 2**).

Athletes with prolonged symptoms require more complex management plans. These athletes may be removed from their activities and social groups, experience difficulties in school and home life, and may suffer from reactive anxiety, depression, and the cardiovascular consequences of prolonged rest. A comprehensive approach to concussion care is vital and aids in smooth RTP and minimizes the effects on school or work. Athletes with multiple concussions or with prolonged PCS should have access to NP testing, psychological intervention, headache management, and expert medical advice.

Given the implications of multiple concussions on future concussion rates and potential for long-term consequences, it is this author's recommendation that athletes with more than 2 to 3 concussions, or with symptoms lasting longer than 2 to 3 weeks, be referred to a physician specializing in concussion, if available. These cases are likely to require further workup, imaging, NP testing, school accommodations, and more involved RTP protocols. Accurate documentation regarding initial activity limitation and eventual RTP guidelines and clearance is a clear part of the current management of concussion, and this is even more critical in states that have passed legislation regarding concussion management.

The future of safe RTP in concussed athletes will ideally involve objective measures of injury and recovery, determination of individual risk based on genetic susceptibility, and a better understanding of the risks for long-term sequelae after multiple concussions. High-quality research is a necessity and will be a responsibility of the overlapping specialties caring for these individuals as concussion management moves forward.

REFERENCES

1. McCrory P, Meeuwisse W, Johnston K, et al. Consensus statement on Concussion in Sport: The 3rd International Conference on Concussion in Sport held in Zurich, November 2008. PM R 2009;1(5):406–20.
2. Protect young athletes. Available at: http://www.cdc.gov/Features/ProtectYoung Athletes/. Accessed January 5, 2011.
3. Langlois JA, Rutland-Brown W, Wald MM. The epidemiology and impact of traumatic brain injury: a brief overview. J Head Trauma Rehabil 2006;21(5):375–8.
4. Heads up: concussion in youth sports. Available at: http://www.cdc.gov/concussion/HeadsUp/youth.html. Accessed January 5, 2011.
5. Available at: http://www.cdc.gov/media/pressrel/braini1.htm. Accessed January 5, 2011.
6. Yard EE, Comstock RD. Compliance with return to play guidelines following concussion in US high school athletes, 2005-2008. Brain Inj 2009;23(11): 888–98.
7. Giza CC, Hovda DA. The neurometabolic cascade of concussion. J Athl Train 2001;36(3):228–35.

8. Giza CC, DiFiori JP. Pathophysiology of sports-related concussion. Sports Health: A Multidisciplinary Approach 2011;3(1):46–51.
9. Tavazzi B, Vagnozzi R, Signoretti S, et al. Temporal window of metabolic brain vulnerability to concussions: oxidative and nitrosative stresses–part II. Neurosurgery 2007;61(2):390–5 [discussion: 395–6].
10. Vagnozzi R, Tavazzi B, Signoretti S, et al. Temporal window of metabolic brain vulnerability to concussions: mitochondrial-related impairment–part I. Neurosurgery 2007;61(2):379–88 [discussion: 388–9].
11. Signoretti S, Vagnozzi R, Tavazzi B, et al. Biochemical and neurochemical sequelae following mild traumatic brain injury: summary of experimental data and clinical implications. Neurosurg Focus 2010;29(5):E1.
12. Daneshvar DH, Nowinski CJ, McKee AC, et al. The epidemiology of sport-related concussion. Clin Sports Med 2011;30(1):1–17, vii.
13. Agel J, Evans TA, Dick R, et al. Descriptive epidemiology of collegiate men's soccer injuries: National Collegiate Athletic Association Injury Surveillance System, 1988-1989 through 2002-2003. J Athl Train 2007;42(2):270–7.
14. Dick R, Ferrara MS, Agel J, et al. Descriptive epidemiology of collegiate men's football injuries: National Collegiate Athletic Association Injury Surveillance System, 1988-1989 through 2003-2004. J Athl Train 2007;42(2):221–33.
15. Dick R, Putukian M, Agel J, et al. Descriptive epidemiology of collegiate women's soccer injuries: National Collegiate Athletic Association Injury Surveillance System, 1988-1989 through 2002-2003. J Athl Train 2007;42(2):278–85.
16. McCrea M, Guskiewicz KM, Marshall SW, et al. Acute effects and recovery time following concussion in collegiate football players: the NCAA Concussion Study. JAMA 2003;290(19):2556–63.
17. McCrea M, Guskiewicz K, Randolph C, et al. Effects of a symptom-free waiting period on clinical outcome and risk of reinjury after sport-related concussion. Neurosurgery 2009;65(5):876–82 [discussion: 882–3].
18. Lincoln AE, Caswell SV, Almquist JL, et al. Trends in concussion incidence in high school sports: a prospective 11-year study. Am J Sports Med 2011;39(5):958–63.
19. McCrory P, Meeuwisse W, Johnston K, et al. Consensus statement on Concussion in Sport: the 3rd International Conference on Concussion in Sport held in Zurich, November 2008. Br J Sports Med 2009;43(Suppl 1):i76–90.
20. Cantu RC, Guskiewicz K, Register-Mihalik JK. A retrospective clinical analysis of moderate to severe athletic concussions. PM R 2010;2(12):1088–93.
21. Guskiewicz KM, McCrea M, Marshall SW, et al. Cumulative effects associated with recurrent concussion in collegiate football players: the NCAA Concussion Study. JAMA 2003;290(19):2549–55.
22. Collins MW, Lovell MR, Iverson GL, et al. Cumulative effects of concussion in high school athletes. Neurosurgery 2002;51(5):1175–9 [discussion: 1180–1].
23. Chen JK, Johnston KM, Petrides M, et al. Neural substrates of symptoms of depression following concussion in male athletes with persisting postconcussion symptoms. Arch Gen Psychiatry 2008;65(1):81–9.
24. Kashluba S, Casey JE, Paniak C. Evaluating the utility of ICD-10 diagnostic criteria for postconcussion syndrome following mild traumatic brain injury. J Int Neuropsychol Soc 2006;12(1):111–8.
25. Bryant RA. Disentangling mild traumatic brain injury and stress reactions. N Engl J Med 2008;358(5):525–7.
26. Guskiewicz KM, Bruce SL, Cantu RC, et al. National athletic trainers' association position statement: management of sport-related concussion. J Athl Train 2004; 39(3):280–97.

27. Kutcher JS, Giza CC, Alessi AG. Clinical practice reference sheet for clinicians. American Academy of Neurology; 2010. Available at: http://www.aan.com/globals/axon/assets/8315.pdf. Accessed August 8, 2011.
28. 2010-2011 Sports Medicine Handbook. Indianapolis (IN): NCAA; 2011. Available at: http://www.ncaapublications.com/p-4203-2010-2011-sports-medicine-handbook.aspx. Accessed August 8, 2011.
29. Available at: http://www.nfl.com/news/story?confirm=true&id=09000d5d814a9ecd&template=with-video-with-comments. Accessed January 19, 2011.
30. Wetjen NM, Pichelmann MA, Atkinson JL. Second impact syndrome: concussion and second injury brain complications. J Am Coll Surg 2010;211(4):553–7.
31. Cantu RC, Gean AD. Second-impact syndrome and a small subdural hematoma: an uncommon catastrophic result of repetitive head injury with a characteristic imaging appearance. J Neurotrauma 2010;27(9):1557–64.
32. Mori T, Katayama Y, Kawamata T. Acute hemispheric swelling associated with thin subdural hematomas: pathophysiology of repetitive head injury in sports. Acta Neurochir Suppl 2006;96:40–3.
33. McCrory P. Does second impact syndrome exist? Clin J Sport Med 2001;11(3):144–9.
34. Majerske CW, Mihalik JP, Ren D, et al. Concussion in sports: postconcussive activity levels, symptoms, and neurocognitive performance. J Athl Train 2008;43(3):265–74.
35. Leddy JJ, Kozlowski K, Fung M, et al. Regulatory and autoregulatory physiological dysfunction as a primary characteristic of post concussion syndrome: implications for treatment. NeuroRehabilitation 2007;22(3):199–205.
36. Putukian M, Aubry M, McCrory P. Return to play after sports concussion in elite and non-elite athletes? Br J Sports Med 2009;43(Suppl 1):i28–31.
37. Echemendia RJ, Putukian M, Mackin RS, et al. Neuropsychological test performance prior to and following sports-related mild traumatic brain injury. Clin J Sport Med 2001;11(1):23–31.
38. McCrea M, Kelly JP, Randolph C, et al. Immediate neurocognitive effects of concussion. Neurosurgery 2002;50(5):1032–40 [discussion: 1040–2].
39. Moser RS, Iverson GL, Echemendia RJ, et al. Neuropsychological evaluation in the diagnosis and management of sports-related concussion. Arch Clin Neuropsychol 2007;22(8):909–16.
40. Lovell MR, Pardini JE, Welling J, et al. Functional brain abnormalities are related to clinical recovery and time to return-to-play in athletes. Neurosurgery 2007;61(2):352–9 [discussion: 359–60].
41. McClincy MP, Lovell MR, Pardini J, et al. Recovery from sports concussion in high school and collegiate athletes. Brain Inj 2006;20(1):33–9.
42. Iverson GL, Brooks BL, Lovell MR, et al. No cumulative effects for one or two previous concussions. Br J Sports Med 2006;40(1):72–5.
43. Meehan WP 3rd, d'Hemecourt P, Comstock RD. High school concussions in the 2008-2009 academic year: mechanism, symptoms, and management. Am J Sports Med 2010;38(12):2405–9.
44. Jacobson RR. The post-concussional syndrome: physiogenesis, psychogenesis and malingering. An integrative model. J Psychosom Res 1995;39(6):675–93.
45. McLean SA, Kirsch NL, Tan-Schriner CU, et al. Health status, not head injury, predicts concussion symptoms after minor injury. Am J Emerg Med 2009;27(2):182–90.
46. Wood RL. Understanding the 'miserable minority': a diasthesis-stress paradigm for post-concussional syndrome. Brain Inj 2004;18(11):1135–53.
47. Bailey CM, Samples HL, Broshek DK, et al. The relationship between psychological distress and baseline sports-related concussion testing. Clin J Sport Med 2010;20(4):272–7.

48. Kübler-Ross E. On death and dying. 1st Scribner Classics. New York: Scribner Classics; 1997.
49. Walker N, Thatcher J, Lavallee D. Psychological responses to injury in competitive sport: a critical review. J R Soc Promot Health 2007;127(4):174–80.
50. Wiese-bjornstal DM, Smith AM, Shaffer SM, et al. An integrated model of response to sport injury: psychological and sociological dynamics. J Appl Sport Psychol 1998;10(1):46–69.
51. Mainwaring LM, Hutchison M, Bisschop SM, et al. Emotional response to sport concussion compared to ACL injury. Brain Inj 2010;24(4):589–97.
52. Iverson GL. Misdiagnosis of the persistent postconcussion syndrome in patients with depression. Arch Clin Neuropsychol 2006;21(4):303–10.
53. Leddy JJ, Kozlowski K, Donnelly JP, et al. A preliminary study of subsymptom threshold exercise training for refractory post-concussion syndrome. Clin J Sport Med 2010;20(1):21–7.
54. Moser RS, Schatz P, Jordan BD. Prolonged effects of concussion in high school athletes. Neurosurgery 2005;57(2):300–6 [discussion: 300–6].
55. Omalu BI, DeKosky ST, Minster RL, et al. Chronic traumatic encephalopathy in a National Football League player. Neurosurgery 2005;57(1):128–34 [discussion: 128–34].
56. Omalu BI, DeKosky ST, Hamilton RL, et al. Chronic traumatic encephalopathy in a National Football League player: part II. Neurosurgery 2006;59(5):1086–92 [discussion: 1092–3].
57. Omalu BI, Fitzsimmons RP, Hammers J, et al. Chronic traumatic encephalopathy in a professional American wrestler. J Forensic Nurs 2010;6(3):130–6.
58. Omalu BI, Bailes J, Hammers JL, et al. Chronic traumatic encephalopathy, suicides and parasuicides in professional American athletes: the role of the forensic pathologist. Am J Forensic Med Pathol 2010;31(2):130–2.
59. Cantu RC. Chronic traumatic encephalopathy in the National Football League. Neurosurgery 2007;61(2):223–5.
60. McKee AC, Cantu RC, Nowinski CJ, et al. Chronic traumatic encephalopathy in athletes: progressive tauopathy after repetitive head injury. J Neuropathol Exp Neurol 2009;68(7):709–35.
61. Kelly JP, Rosenberg JH. The development of guidelines for the management of concussion in sports. J Head Trauma Rehabil 1998;13(2):53–65.
62. Cantu RC. Return to play guidelines after a head injury. Clin Sports Med 1998;17(1):45–60.
63. Cantu RC. Posttraumatic retrograde and anterograde amnesia: pathophysiology and implications in grading and safe return to play. J Athl Train 2001;36(3):244–8.
64. Cantu RC. Recurrent athletic head injury: risks and when to retire. Clin Sports Med 2003;22(3):593–603, x.
65. McCrory P. 2002 Refshauge Lecture. When to retire after concussion? J Sci Med Sport 2002;5(3):169–82.
66. Practice Guideline from the AAN. AAN Concussion Position Statement: American Academy of Neurology. Available at: http://www.aan.com/globals/axon/assets/7913.pdf. Accessed August 8, 2011.
67. Guskiewicz KM, Weaver NL, Padua DA, et al. Epidemiology of concussion in collegiate and high school football players. Am J Sports Med 2000;28(5):643–50.
68. Zemper ED. Two-year prospective study of relative risk of a second cerebral concussion. Am J Phys Med Rehabil 2003;82(9):653–9.
69. Jotwani V, Harmon KG. Postconcussion syndrome in athletes. Curr Sports Med Rep 2010;9(1):21–6.

70. Collins MW, Grindel SH, Lovell MR, et al. Relationship between concussion and neuropsychological performance in college football players. JAMA 1999; 282(10):964–70.

71. De Beaumont L, Theoret H, Mongeon D, et al. Brain function decline in healthy retired athletes who sustained their last sports concussion in early adulthood. Brain 2009;132(Pt 3):695–708.

72. Covassin T, Elbin R, Kontos A, et al. Investigating baseline neurocognitive performance between male and female athletes with a history of multiple concussion. J Neurol Neurosurg Psychiatry 2010;81(6):597–601.

73. Kuehl MD, Snyder AR, Erickson SE, et al. Impact of prior concussions on health-related quality of life in collegiate athletes. Clin J Sport Med 2010;20(2):86–91.

74. Cantu RC. When to disqualify an athlete after a concussion. Curr Sports Med Rep 2009;8(1):6–7.

75. Schatz P, Moser RS, Covassin T, et al. Early indicators of enduring symptoms in high school athletes with multiple previous concussions. Neurosurgery 2011; 68(6):1562–7.

76. Gavett BE, Stern RA, McKee AC. Chronic traumatic encephalopathy: a potential late effect of sport-related concussive and subconcussive head trauma. Clin Sports Med 2011;30(1):179–88, xi.

77. Guskiewicz KM, Marshall SW, Bailes J, et al. Recurrent concussion and risk of depression in retired professional football players. Med Sci Sports Exerc 2007; 39(6):903–9.

78. Davis G, Marion DW, Le Roux P, et al. Clinics in neurology and neurosurgery–extradural and subdural haematoma. Br J Sports Med 2010;44(16):1139–43.

79. Miele VJ, Bailes JE, Martin NA. Participation in contact or collision sports in athletes with epilepsy, genetic risk factors, structural brain lesions, or history of craniotomy. Neurosurg Focus 2006;21(4):E9.

80. Pearsall AW 4th, Kovaleski JE, Madanagopal SG. Medicolegal issues affecting sports medicine practitioners. Clin Orthop Relat Res 2005;(433):50–7.

81. Practice parameter: the management of concussion in sports (summary statement). Report of the Quality Standards Subcommittee. Neurology 1997;48(3): 581–5.

82. Kelly JP, Nichols JS, Filley CM, et al. Concussion in sports. Guidelines for the prevention of catastrophic outcome. JAMA 1991;266(20):2867–9.

Diagnosis of Concussion: The Role of Imaging Now and in the Future

Brendan J. McCullough, MD, PhD[a,b], Jeffrey G. Jarvik, MD, MPH[b,c],*

KEYWORDS

• Concussion • Mild traumatic brain injury • Youth • Sports
• Computed tomography • Magnetic resonance imaging

Concussion, as defined by the Third International Conference on Concussion in Sport, is a clinical diagnosis (**Box 1**).[1] To paraphrase, "concussion" is a transient neurologic impairment resulting from an impact to the head or body. There is no detectable structural injury on standard neuroimaging studies.

The primary role of neuroimaging in the context of concussion is the exclusion of a more serious, unsuspected diagnosis, such as an epidural hematoma. A small but significant proportion of patients presenting with a clinical history consistent with concussion have an intracranial injury or skull fracture that requires further management. Computed tomography (CT), and to a lesser extent magnetic resonance imaging (MRI), are the imaging modalities of choice for this purpose.

The challenge facing sports-related concussion, particularly in adolescents, is to determine when it is safe to return to play. Athletes with a history of concussion are at increased risk for subsequent concussions compared with teammates.[2] There may also be a temporal window of increased vulnerability during which time even a mild head injury results in a potentially fatal outcome, termed "second impact syndrome."[3] Symptoms are generally used as a guide for return to play decisions,[1,4]

Financial Disclosures: Dr Jarvik is a cofounder and stockholder of PhysioSonics, a consultant for HealthHelp and a consultant for GE Healthcare. Dr McCullough has no financial disclosures. Funding Support: None.
[a] Department of Radiology, University of Washington, 1959 NE Pacific Street, Box 357115, Seattle, WA 98195, USA
[b] Comparative Effectiveness, Cost and Outcomes Research Center, University of Washington, Seattle, WA, USA
[c] Department of Radiology, Neurological Surgery, and Health Services, University of Washington, Seattle, WA, USA
* Corresponding author. Department of Radiology, Harborview Medical Center, 325 Ninth Avenue, Box 359728, Seattle, WA 98104–2499.
E-mail address: jarvikj@uw.edu

Phys Med Rehabil Clin N Am 22 (2011) 635–652
doi:10.1016/j.pmr.2011.08.005
1047-9651/11/$ – see front matter © 2011 Elsevier Inc. All rights reserved.

Box 1
Definition of concussion according to the Zurich Consensus statement from the Third International Conference on Concussion in Sport (November, 2008)

Concussion is defined as a complex pathophysiologic process affecting the brain, induced by traumatic biomechanical forces. Several common features that incorporate clinical, pathologic, and biomechanical injury constructs that may be used in defining the nature of a concussive head injury include:

1. Concussion may be caused either by a direct blow to the head, face, neck, or elsewhere on the body with an "impulsive" force transmitted to the head.
2. Concussion typically results in the rapid onset of short-lived impairment of neurologic function that resolves spontaneously.
3. Concussion may result in neuropathologic changes but the acute clinical symptoms largely reflect a functional disturbance rather than a structural injury.
4. Concussion results in a graded set of clinical symptoms that may or may not involve loss of consciousness. Resolution of the clinical and cognitive symptoms typically follows a sequential course; however, it is important to note that in a small percentage of cases postconcussive symptoms may be prolonged.
5. No abnormality on standard structural neuroimaging studies is seen in concussion.

Data from McCrory P, Meeuwisse W, Johnston K, et al. Consensus Statement on Concussion in Sport: the 3rd International Conference on Concussion in Sport held in Zurich, November 2008. Br J Sports Med 2009;43(Suppl 1):i76–90.

---

but these may not be sensitive enough or there may be incentive or social pressure for an athlete to deny symptoms to play. There is a potential role for new, more sensitive imaging techniques directed at the underlying pathophysiology of concussion to help guide rehabilitation and return to play decisions.

This article first focuses on the current role of imaging for the exclusion of unsuspected intracranial injuries in the clinical context of concussion. Emerging techniques are then discussed in the context of the current understanding of the molecular and cellular pathophysiology underlying concussion. Throughout this review, evidence pertaining to adolescent sports-related concussion is considered primarily. As our understanding of the pathophysiology of concussion evolves, it is clear that concussion represents the mild end of the spectrum of traumatic brain injury (TBI) and there is significant overlap between the terms "concussion" and "mild TBI" (mTBI). As such, evidence from mTBI or more severe injuries is also considered when appropriate.

DIAGNOSING CONCUSSION: EXCLUDING A MORE SEVERE INJURY
Epidemiology of Intracranial Injuries

The Centers for Disease Control and Prevention estimates that 135,000 persons aged 5 to 18 years are treated for sports-related TBI in hospital emergency departments in the United States annually.[5] Most patients will have suffered only a mild head injury and are neurologically normal on presentation, consistent with the diagnosis of concussion. However, a small but significant proportion of these harbor intracranial injuries evident on neuroimaging that require further management.

The frequency of traumatic intracranial injuries in adolescents after minor, sports-related head trauma is not known. Multiple studies have measured the rates of intracranial injuries (including skull fractures) on CT and subsequent neurosurgical interventions in patients presenting to emergency departments after minor head injury and with a normal Glasgow Coma Scale (GCS) score of 15 (**Table 1**).[6–12] In the general population, rates of detected intracranial injuries ranged from 3.3% to 34% and rates of intervention, usually neurosurgical, ranged from 0.3% to 1%. Studies involving only pediatric patients tended to have higher rates of intracranial abnormalities and interventions.[8,10] Two meta-analyses concluded the overall rates of intracranial injury are approximately 5% to 8%, rates of neurosurgical intervention are less than 1%, and approximately 1 in 1000 patients will die.[13,14]

It should be noted that although sports-related head injuries were included in these studies, the predominant mechanism of injury was motor vehicle collision, likely exposing the patient to greater forces than that seen in sports. The two pediatric studies required a "nontrivial" or "high-risk" mechanism.[8,10] Furthermore, several studies included only patients with head injuries resulting in loss of consciousness. As such, these studies are complicated by selection bias, likely overestimating the true rate of unsuspected intracranial injury in patients presenting with mild head trauma. However, the devastating potential of these injuries makes even a low rate significant.

Radiography

Plain radiographs of the skull have been used in the assessment of head injury to identify fractures as a marker for intracranial injury.[15–17] The advantage of radiographs is that they are cheap and ubiquitously available. Their great disadvantage is their lack of sensitivity, and since the advent of CT, skull radiographs have been essentially abandoned.

The usefulness of plain radiography of the skull in patients presenting with concussion is extremely limited. Radiographs can identify skull fractures, but not underlying brain injury. Patients may have a fracture without underlying intracranial injury or they may have a serious intracranial injury without fracture. Teasdale and colleagues[15] examined 8051 patients, 3491 children (2–14 years of age) and 4560 adults, who presented to Scottish emergency departments between 1974 and 1984 with a head injury and a GCS of 15. Of the patients with clinically diagnosed, intracranial hemorrhage requiring neurosurgical intervention, only 18 (53%) of 34 children and 86 (71%) of 121 adults had skull fractures diagnosed by radiographs. Furthermore, skull fractures were detected in 61 (41%) of 147 of adults and 48 (73%) of 66 of children who did not require intervention. Thus, skull radiographs may be falsely reassuring if they are normal or may lead to unnecessary intervention if they are abnormal.

Other studies have shown similar results, including a meta-analysis that estimated the sensitivity of skull radiographs for the detection of intracranial hemorrhage in minor

Table 1
Epidemiology of unsuspected intracranial injuries with normal GCS score

Study, Year	Ages (Mean)	No.	LOC (%)	Positive CT	Intervention
Haydel & Shembekar,[8] 2003	5–17 (13)	175	100	14 (8%)	1 (0.6%)
Simon et al,[10] 2001	<16 (7)	499	46[a]	120 (24%)	5 (1%)
Stein & Ross,[6] 1992	NA (NA)	1117	100	73 (13.2%)	NA
Haydel et al,[9] 2000	≥3 (36)	1429	100	93 (6.5%)	6 (0.4%)
Smits et al,[12] 2005	≥16 (41[a])	2462	61[a]	185 (7.5%)	10 (0.4%)
Thiruppathy & Muthukumar,[11] 2004	All (NA)	285	40	98 (34%)	18 (6%)
Nagy et al,[7] 1999	All (34)	1170	100	39 (3.3%)	4 (0.3%)

Abbreviations: GCS, Glasgow Coma Scale score; LOC, loss of consciousness; NA, not available.
[a] Statistic calculated from entire study sample, including patients with GCS 13–15.

head injury to be 38%, using CT of the head as the reference standard.[16,17] As a result, current guidelines for the management of pediatric or sports-related concussions ignore or discourage the use of radiography as a test for intracranial injury in favor of CT.[1,4,18–20]

Computed Tomography

CT is the imaging modality of choice for initial screening of patients presenting with a history of mild head injury to exclude a more serious intracranial injury. Compared with standard MRI, CT is more widely available in terms of both locations and hours of operation,[21] and it is significantly faster, requiring only seconds for a head CT. Aside from minimizing the time the patient is in the scanner, a faster examination limits the potential for motion artifact, a significant consideration in disoriented patients or young children.

Modern CT scanners move the patient past a rotating x-ray tube (<1 s per rotation), acquiring a helical dataset of x-ray attenuation measurements. Multidetector CT scanners have multiple rows of detectors (eg, 4, 16, 64, 128, and so forth, sometimes referred to as "slices") along the z-axis (craniocaudal), allowing greater coverage per rotation, higher resolution, and faster scan times, although generally at a cost of more radiation exposure.[22] A computer processes the dataset and generates gray-scale representations of x-ray attenuation. Attenuation is measured in Hounsfield units (HU), where water is set at 0 and greater attenuation (eg, bone or contrast material) results in positive values and lesser attenuation (eg, air) results in negative values (−1000 HU for air).[23]

Modern CT scanners can achieve a resolution of fractions of a millimeter in all planes, although images of the head are most commonly reconstructed in the axial plane with a slice thickness of 5 mm. The original dataset can often be used to create reformations in any plane or even three-dimensional representations.

CT is most sensitive for the detection of acute hemorrhage and fractures (**Fig. 1**). In the brain, white and gray matter measure approximately 40 and 35 HU, respectively, whereas acute hemorrhage measures 50 to 90 HU. Multiplanar and three-dimensional reformations increase sensitivity for fractures and lesions parallel to the standard, axial plane, such as thin subdural hematomas near the skull apex (**Figs. 2** and **3**).

Ionizing Radiation

CT uses ionizing radiation (x-rays), which carries its own risks and deserves mention. The energy imparted in biologic tissues can be harmful in two ways. First, sufficiently high radiation exposure directly kills cells, resulting in skin erythema (burn), epilation (hair loss), or necrosis. These effects are threshold dependent and the radiation dose needed for even minor skin effects is extremely uncommon with CT.

More relevant to CT are stochastic effects, representing the likelihood of radiation exposure to induce cancer at the molecular level. These effects are generally assumed to be linearly related to dose and not threshold dependent: a single photon has the theoretical potential to induce a cancer-causing mutation. Effective dose (ED), measured in sieverts (Sv), attempts to estimate this risk by taking into account absorbed radiation dose (measured in gray [Gy]) and the radiosensitivity of the exposed organs.[23,24]

A routine head CT has an ED of approximately 2 mSv (range, 0.3–6 mSv).[25,26] **Table 2** compares the median ED of common medical imaging tests and equivalent exposure from naturally occurring background radiation and a two-view chest radiograph series. For a variety of reasons, ED also increases with decreasing patient age.[22] King and colleagues[26] reported EDs for a head CT at a regional children's hospital of 1.7, 2.1, and 2.4 mSv in age groups of 10 to 14, 4 to 9, and 0 to 3 years, respectively.

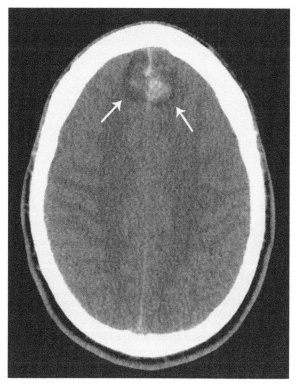

Fig. 1. A 16-year-old male football player injured landing on the back of his head after diving for a pass. Patient had no loss of consciousness and a GCS score of 15. He was originally seen at an outside hospital and sent home without imaging and a diagnosis of concussion. He represented the following morning because of persistent headache and emesis. Axial CT image demonstrates bifrontal hemorrhagic contusions (*arrows*) with a small amount of subarachnoid hemorrhage along the anterior falx.

Estimates for the lifetime risk of developing cancer from radiation exposure are challenging with medical imaging because the doses are so low. The lifetime risk of developing a solid cancer in the absence of exposure from medical imaging is estimated to be 45.5% in men and 36.9% in women. A 2-mSv head CT is estimated to increase this risk by 16 per 100,000 (0.016%) in men and 26 per 100,000 (0.026%) in women.[27] **Table 3** gives complete estimates for cancers and related deaths.

When to Image

Current guidelines for the use of CT in the context of sports-related or pediatric concussion are based on expert opinion and recommend imaging when a structural, intracranial injury is clinically suspected.[1,18,19] No prospective studies have been performed to evaluate these guidelines.

Several studies have attempted to devise and validate clinical decision rules for the use of CT in minor head injury in the general population. The two most established of these are the New Orleans Criteria and the Canadian Head CT Rule.[9,12,28] However, the applicability of these recommendations to adolescent sports-related concussion is not clear. Ultimately, the decision to perform a CT in the context of sports-related concussion is a clinical decision based on the risks of a serious, underlying intracranial injury or skull fracture versus the risks of harm from radiation.

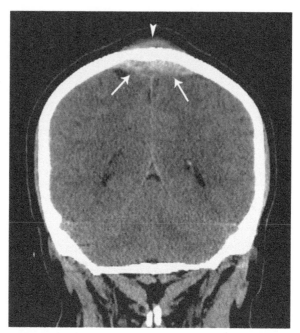

Fig. 2. A 23-year-old man found unconscious after a fall from a skateboard. Coronal reformation of CT best demonstrates subdural hematoma at the skull vertex (*arrows*). Subgaleal hematoma is present (*arrowhead*).

Magnetic Resonance Imaging

MRI uses a strong magnetic field and radiofrequency pulses of energy to excite and detect hydrogen protons. Most importantly, it does not use ionizing radiation. A typical examination involves multiple sequences that generally must be acquired

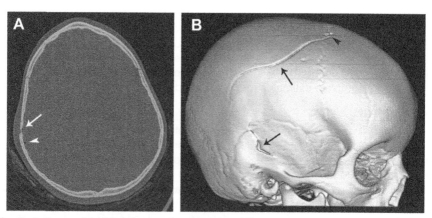

Fig. 3. A 6-year-old girl fell out of a window while jumping on a bed. Standard two-dimensional axial CT image (*A*) demonstrates mildly displaced right parietal bone fracture (*arrow*) with tiny adjacent pneumocephalus (*arrowhead*). Course of the fracture (*arrows*) is easily visualized on three-dimensional reformation (*B*) and extension into coronal suture is evident (*arrowhead*).

Table 2
Effective doses (mSv) of common medical imaging examinations and equivalents

Examination	ED (IQR)	Background Radiation	Chest Radiographs
Head CT	2 (2–3)	8 months	30
Neck CT	4 (3–6)	16 months	55
Chest CT	8 (5–11)	32 months	117
Abdomen-pelvis CT with contrast	16 (11–20)	64 months	234

Background radiation is assumed to be 3 mSv/yr in the United States.
Abbreviation: IQR, interquartile range.
Data from Huda W, Vance A. Patient radiation doses from adult and pediatric CT. AJR Am J Roentgenol 2007;188(2):540–6; and Smith-Bindman R, Lipson J, Marcus R, et al. Radiation dose associated with common computed tomography examinations and the associated lifetime attributable risk of cancer. Arch Intern Med 2009;169(22):2078–86.

sequentially. The plane of imaging is set for each sequence and usually includes some combination of axial, coronal, and sagittal planes of various sequences. Some sequences may be acquired in a volumetric manner, allowing multiplanar reformations to be performed.

The primary sequences are T1- and T2-weighted. These reflect different measures of relaxation of hydrogen protons to their low-energy state. Fluid is dark on T1-weighted images and bright on T2-weighted images. Fluid-attenuated inversion recovery (FLAIR) is an additional T2-weighted sequence in which the signal from cerebrospinal fluid is nullified, enhancing lesion conspicuity, such as edema.[23,29] Diffusion-weighted and T2*-weighted imaging is also commonly performed in the context of trauma and is further described later.

MRI is exquisitely sensitive for parenchymal lesions because these usually involve some degree of edema and are hyperintense on T2-weighted or FLAIR images (**Fig. 4**). Acute hemorrhage (1–3 days) is hypointense on T2-weighted images because of the paramagnetic effect of the iron contained within the hemoglobin. This paramagnetic effect is especially evident on the gradient recalled echo T2*-weighted sequence, which is similar to T2 but is more susceptible to irregularities in the magnetic field. On this sequence, blood products result in complete signal dropout and there is also "blooming," making even punctate hemorrhages, as seen with diffuse axonal injury (DAI), stand out (**Fig. 5**). Susceptibility-weighted imaging is a variation of this technique that has been described and is reported to have even greater sensitivity for blood products.[30] As blood products evolve, they undergo predictable changes in their appearance on T1- and T2-weighted images, allowing estimation of their age.

Table 3
Lifetime attributable risk estimates for solid cancer from a head CT per 100,000 individuals

	All Solid Cancer		Leukemia	
	Male	Female	Male	Female
Cases in absence of exposure	45,500	36,900	830	590
Cases attributable to exposure	16	26	2	1.4
Deaths in absence of exposure	22,100	17,500	710	530
Deaths attributable to exposure	8.2	12.2	1.4	1

Based on BEIR VII for a 2-mSv exposure.[27]

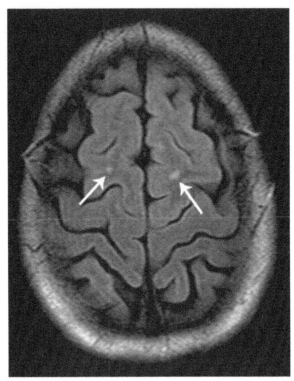

Fig. 4. A 21-year-old woman struck on the head by an assailant. CT scan at the time was normal (not shown). MRI was performed because of persistent headache and subjective neurocognitive impairment 5 weeks after the injury. Axial FLAIR image demonstrates focal areas of increased signal (*arrows*) in the paramedian subcortical white matter of bilateral posterior frontal lobes.

Sensitivity of CT Versus MRI

Multiple studies have demonstrated MRI to be more sensitive for the detection of intracranial injuries than CT, with the exception of subarachnoid hemorrhages and fractures.[31–34] For intracranial injuries severe enough to require neurosurgical intervention, however, CT and MRI are equivalent.[31,32] CT has been shown in a meta-analysis to be nearly 100% sensitive for the detection of life-threatening injuries.[35]

The differences in sensitivity are best demonstrated in the study by Lee and colleagues[33] using essentially modern equipment (**Table 4**). This study prospectively compared 36 adult patients with mild TBI (GCS 13–15) using conventional CT with 5-mm axial slices and 3-T MRI using three different sequences (including three-dimensional and T2*-weighted sequences) with 1- to 3-mm slice thickness. MRI showed greater sensitivity in detecting intraparenchymal injuries, particularly DAI and nonhemorrhagic contusions. Subdural hematomas were also detected more frequently with MRI, but this may be at least partially caused by multiple planes of imaging, which is available on modern CT scanners but not used in this study. Of note, subarachnoid hemorrhage was detected more frequently with CT. This study did not include cranial fractures, which CT is significantly better at revealing.[31]

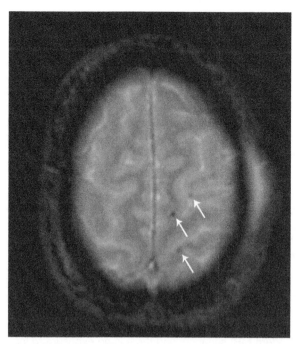

Fig. 5. A 16-year-old girl injured in a high-speed motor vehicle crash. Axial gradient recalled echo T2* image demonstrates foci of signal drop-out (*arrows*) in the subcortical white matter of the posterior left frontal lobe, consistent with petechial hemorrhage and diffuse axonal injury.

Table 4
Imaging findings in 36 adult patients with mild traumatic brain injury

	CT	MRI
Abnormal	23	27
Epidural hematoma	4	3
Subdural hematoma	6	11
Subarachnoid hemorrhage	8	2
Intraventricular hemorrhage	1	0
Intraparenchymal injury	18	27
DAI		
Hemorrhagic	8	17
Nonhemorrhagic	0	4
Contusions		
Hemorrhagic	12	17
Nonhemorrhagic	1	4

Abbreviation: DAI, diffuse axonal injury.

Data from Lee H, Wintermark M, Gean AD, et al. Focal lesions in acute mild traumatic brain injury and neurocognitive outcome: CT versus 3T MRI. J Neurotrauma 2008;25(9):1049–56.

DIFFERENTIATING CONCUSSIONS: EMERGING TECHNOLOGIES
A Molecular and Cellular Understanding of Concussion

Although the mechanism underlying concussion is controversial, it is generally believed to result from shearing stress caused by rotational or angular acceleration and differences in stiffness of neural elements, namely gray and white matter.[36,37] As the shearing stress increases, there is axonal stretching and disruption of cell membranes. Indiscriminate ion flux across the membrane ensues with concomitant loss of ionic and neurochemical homeostasis. With minor injuries, these changes are transient and self-limited. More severe injuries may result in longer-lasting or permanent structural injury to axons.[38]

Shearing injury, termed DAI or traumatic axonal injury, has been well described on MRI and CT in TBI generally as petechial hemorrhages or hyperintense foci in the white matter on fluid-sensitive MRI sequences.[39] Studies have also shown the burden of DAI on MRI was associated with worse outcomes in TBI.[40,41] However, there is increasing evidence that suggests DAI also occurs in mTBI and concussion, but it is below the detection threshold of modern CT and MRI.[39,42]

More sensitive imaging techniques are currently being developed to measure these molecular and microstructural injuries. Although these techniques are not routinely used clinically, they have demonstrated the ability to detect regional abnormalities of neurometabolites (magnetic resonance spectroscopy [MRS]), microstructural axonal injury (diffusion tensor imaging [DTI]), and abnormal cortical activation patterns (functional MRI [fMRI]) after concussion. Moreover, the necessary hardware already exists in most modern MRI scanners and there is no exposure to ionizing radiation.

Magnetic Resonance Spectroscopy

MRI measures the signal derived from the relaxation of hydrogen protons in a magnetic field. Most of this signal arises from water and lipids, the predominant hydrogen-containing molecules in tissue. ^{1}H MRS focuses on other, less concentrated hydrogen proton-containing molecules. The resulting signal is analyzed as a spectrum of chemical shifts and common molecules can be identified as characteristic peaks in the spectrum (**Fig. 6**). Metabolites are generally normalized to creatine (Cr), a marker of metabolism that is relatively stable.[30]

Several studies have demonstrated a reduction in the concentration of N-acetylaspartate (NAA) after sports-related concussion. NAA is synthesized by mitochondria of neurons; reductions in NAA are associated with neuronal or axonal injury or loss.[43] Henry and colleagues[44] studied 12 intercollegiate varsity athletes who had sustained a "sports concussion" (GCS 13–15) within 6 days of imaging. Compared with healthy, age-matched controls, NAA/Cr levels were significantly reduced in the primary motor cortex and to a lesser extent in the dorsolateral prefrontal cortex (DLPC) in concussed athletes. NAA/Cr in the primary motor cortex was also shown to be negatively correlated with self-reported symptom scores in concussed athletes: greater drops in NAA/Cr were associated with worse symptoms.

Vagnozzi and colleagues[45] also found reductions in NAA/Cr in the subcortical white matter of the frontal lobes in 10 concussed athletes compared with healthy, age-matched controls. In this study, the authors performed serial MRS examinations at 3, 15, and 30 days postinjury and demonstrated normalization of NAA/Cr by 30 days. Of note, self-reported symptoms had resolved by the first examination. Furthermore, three additional subjects were studied who sustained a second concussion before the 15-day scan. NAA/Cr levels remained depressed disproportionately longer in these subjects, normalizing at 45 days from the initial concussion. The authors

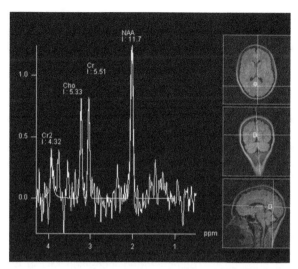

Fig. 6. MR spectroscopy was performed in a 30-year-old woman, nontrauma patient to investigate focus of abnormally increased T2/FLAIR signal in the medial posterior cingulate gyrus. Spectrogram (*left*) demonstrates peaks corresponding to common neurometabolites (labeled). NAA/Cr ratio is mildly reduced, in this case because of a low-grade astrocytoma. Multiplanar FLAIR localization images (*right*) show the voxel used for MR spectroscopy measurement.

suggested this may reflect a temporal window during which the brain is more vulnerable to repeat injury akin to second impact syndrome.

Additional groups have examined patients with more severe TBI and also demonstrated significant reductions in NAA/Cr.[46–49] Decreased glutamate, an excitatory neurotransmitter and associated with excitotoxicity, and increased choline, a marker of membrane turnover, inflammation, or myelination, have also been show to be associated with head injury.[44,49]

The results of these studies suggest that MRS is a sensitive measure of neurometabolic abnormalities after sports-related concussion. Moreover, changes in neurometabolite concentrations can be followed to recovery. However, these studies are based on small numbers of subjects and should be viewed as preliminary. The comparisons reported were statistical differences in means between injured and uninjured groups. Variability among individual subjects suggests that applying these findings on an individual basis may be more difficult.[45,47]

Diffusion Tensor Imaging

Diffusion-weighted imaging has become commonplace as a means of early detection of brain ischemia in stroke and DAI.[39,50] The underlying principle is that water molecules, primarily extracellular, diffuse freely because of Brownian motion. Water molecules in ischemic brain tissue, however, are restricted in their motion, and diffusion-weighted imaging can detect this restriction.[50]

DTI takes this concept further by measuring the magnitude of water diffusivity in each orthogonal axis (x, y, and z) on a voxel-by-voxel basis. The result is a tensor comprised of three orthogonal vectors (eigenvectors). A voxel containing water molecules without any diffusion restriction is isotropic, having eigenvectors of equal magnitude. The tightly packed bundles of axons and myelin within white matter tracts, however, tend to restrict the diffusivity of water molecules in directions perpendicular to the tract. As such, the eigenvector along the tract is significantly larger than that perpendicular to the tract, and this asymmetry in vectors is termed "anisotropy." Anisotropy is quantified as fractional anisotropy (FA), which is represented by a value between 0 and 1, where 0 is completely isotropic and 1 is completely anisotropic. Typical FA values of white matter in the corpus callosum are approximately 0.6 to 0.8. Alternatively, the directional diffusivity can be quantified as mean diffusivity (MD), representing the average of the eigenvectors. In this case, restricting diffusion (in one or more directions) results in decreased MD. Furthermore, because the predominant direction of water diffusivity can be measured on a voxel-by-voxel basis, white matter tracts can be inferred and depicted with color-coded three-dimensional models, termed "tractography" (**Fig. 7**). Typically, an FA threshold of approximately 0.2 is used for directionality.[50,51]

Considering DTI in patients with mTBI, two patterns have emerged in the literature. First, several studies have shown decreased FA or increased MD in mTBI patients compared with age-matched, healthy controls, indicating loss of directional diffusivity (ie, anisotropy) and suggesting microstructural disruption of white matter.[52–55] Of these, Cubon and colleagues[52] demonstrated increased MD in college students with sports-related concussion (GCS 15). The other studies demonstrated decreased FA and increased MD (when reported) in patients with mTBI, but these studies tended to use patients with more severe injuries (GCS 13–15 or abnormalities on conventional MRI). Of note, in all cases the concussed subjects were imaged at least 1 month after injury and had persistent symptoms.

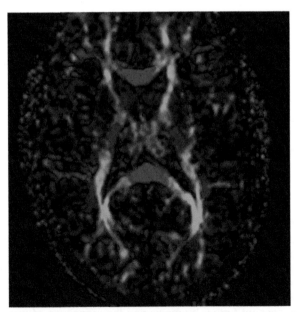

Fig. 7. A 15-year-old football player diagnosed with three concussions from hard tackles sustained during the prior year. CT was performed after the most recent concussion at an outside hospital and was reportedly normal. DTI was performed for further evaluation. Axial tractography image demonstrates white matter tracts color-coded by orientation. No abnormality was identified.

Other studies have demonstrated seemingly contradictory increases in FA in patients after mTBI compared with controls.[56,57] These patients were imaged sooner after their injury (no one beyond 21 days), unlike the previously mentioned studies. The authors suggest this may be caused by acute axonal injury resulting in an overall reduction in diffusivity akin to cytotoxic edema. As such, decreased FA in mTBI may represent chronic structural injuries and correlate with postconcussion symptoms.

As with MRS, these studies are based on small numbers and should be viewed as preliminary. The use of MD versus FA is not clearly defined because the more sensitive measure varied by study. The location of the injury also varied by study, which likely reflects the diffuse nature of microscopic DAI, but random differences could be caused by statistical chance given the large number of voxels sampled. Finally, there seems to be significant variation among subjects, especially with age,[52] which also makes applying these measures on an individual basis difficult.

Functional Magnetic Resonance Imaging

Activation of a particular population of neurons results in increased metabolic demands and compensatory local hyperperfusion. This hyperperfusion, however, exceeds the oxygen demands of the tissue and the net result is excess oxygenated hemoglobin relative to deoxygenated. This difference can be measured using the technique termed "blood oxygen level dependent" (BOLD) fMRI. To accentuate the differences, this test is usually used while a patient completes neurocognitive tasks, thus placing increased demand on the brain, and differences in local perfusion are measured in real time.[58]

Several groups have used fMRI to demonstrate abnormal activation patterns in the brains of athletes after concussion or mTBI.[59–62] Chen and colleagues[60] performed BOLD fMRI in 16 athletes who had sustained at least one concussion and eight age-matched, normal controls. Of note, the time since the last concussion ranged from 1 to 14 months and all but one of the concussed athletes had persistent, post-concussive symptoms. Participants were asked to perform a task designed to test working memory and known to cause consistent and reliable activation of the DLPC on BOLD fMRI. Concussed and control groups performed equivalently on this task. Whereas the control group demonstrated the expected DLPC activation, the concussed group showed significantly lower activation in this location. Moreover, several concussed subjects demonstrated activation during the task outside of the DLPC that was not seen in controls. A subsequent study by the same group with nine symptomatic, concussed athletes confirmed these findings, leading the authors to suggest that the additional foci of activation elsewhere in the brain represent a compensatory mechanism for the lost DLPC activity, allowing the brain to maintain performance on the task.[59] McAllister and colleagues[63] reported similar results in a more heterogeneous group of 18 patients with mTBI (GCS 13–15), eight of which were sports-related. In their subsequent study, Chen and colleagues[59] also showed that activation patterns returned to normal in those subjects whose symptoms resolved.

Lovell and colleagues[62] performed BOLD fMRI in 28 concussed high school athletes (mean age 16.6 years) and 13 age-matched controls while subjects completed the N-back task, a commonly used test of working memory. They found that the severity of postconcussive symptoms in concussed subjects was correlated with activation of the posterior parietal cortex. Additionally, activation of an area of the medial premotor cortex (Brodmann area 6) correlated with longer recovery, as measured by return to play.

These studies suggest abnormal activation patterns of the brain may represent a compensatory mechanism to injury in the normal processing pathways and that fMRI can detect this abnormality. Furthermore, postconcussion symptoms may be the result of the brain needing to use these compensatory, and presumably less efficient, pathways. However, intersubject variability again makes this technique difficult to apply prospectively to individual patients.

Other Imaging Modalities

Several other imaging modalities have been used to evaluate TBI, although generally for injuries more severe than concussion. Positron emission tomography uses radio-labeled fluoro-2-deoxyglucose to measure brain metabolic activity. Several groups have demonstrated persistent symptoms are associated with decreased fluoro-2-deoxyglucose avidity and hence decreased metabolism after TBI.[64–67] Single-photon emission computed tomography uses a radioisotope to measure cerebral blood flow. Metabolic activity is inferred, similar to fMRI. Several studies have also used this technique in patients with mTBI and have shown decreased regional perfusion.[65,68,69] These techniques, however, are relatively costly and require the use of intravenous injection of radioactive isotopes. They remain experimental and are not commonly used or recommended because of the necessary radiation exposure.

SUMMARY

Currently, the role of neuroimaging in adolescent sports-related concussion is limited to excluding more serious, unsuspected intracranial injuries. CT is the imaging modality of choice because it is fast, readily available, and nearly 100% sensitive for injuries that may require intervention. MRI is an alternative to CT that is more sensitive to nonhemorrhagic parenchymal injuries and avoids the use of ionizing radiation. Ultimately, the decision to image is a balance between the risks of an unsuspected, potentially life-threatening injury and the risks of radiation exposure.

Several emerging neuroimaging techniques have shown promise as sensitive measures of the metabolic and microstructural injuries underlying concussion or mTBI. Differences in regional neurometabolites, particularly decreased NAA, have been demonstrated with MRS. Acute and chronic changes in water diffusivity have been shown in white matter tracts with DTI. Finally, fMRI has revealed abnormal, likely compensatory, neurocognitive activation patterns after concussion. In the future, these emerging techniques may be used as tools for directing rehabilitation after concussion and aiding in the decision of when it is safe for an athlete to return to play.

REFERENCES

1. McCrory P, Meeuwisse W, Johnston K, et al. Consensus Statement on Concussion in Sport: the 3rd International Conference on Concussion in Sport held in Zurich, November 2008. Br J Sports Med 2009;43(Suppl 1):i76–90.
2. Guskiewicz KM, McCrea M, Marshall SW, et al. Cumulative effects associated with recurrent concussion in collegiate football players: the NCAA Concussion Study. JAMA 2003;290(19):2549–55.
3. Wetjen NM, Pichelmann MA, Atkinson JL. Second impact syndrome: concussion and second injury brain complications. J Am Coll Surg 2010;211(4):553–7.
4. Halstead ME, Walter KD. American Academy of Pediatrics. Clinical report: sport-related concussion in children and adolescents. Pediatrics 2010;126(3):597–615.
5. Centers for Disease Control and Prevention (CDC). Nonfatal traumatic brain injuries from sports and recreation activities—United States, 2001-2005. MMWR Morb Mortal Wkly Rep 2007;56(29):733–7.

6. Stein SC, Ross SE. Mild head injury: a plea for routine early CT scanning. J Trauma 1992;33(1):11–3.
7. Nagy KK, Joseph KT, Krosner SM, et al. The utility of head computed tomography after minimal head injury. J Trauma 1999;46(2):268–70.
8. Haydel MJ, Shembekar AD. Prediction of intracranial injury in children aged five years and older with loss of consciousness after minor head injury due to nontrivial mechanisms. Ann Emerg Med 2003;42(4):507–14.
9. Haydel MJ, Preston CA, Mills TJ, et al. Indications for computed tomography in patients with minor head injury. N Engl J Med 2000;343(2):100–5.
10. Simon B, Letourneau P, Vitorino E, et al. Pediatric minor head trauma: indications for computed tomographic scanning revisited. J Trauma 2001;51(2):231–7 [discussion: 237–8].
11. Thiruppathy SP, Muthukumar N. Mild head injury: revisited. Acta Neurochir (Wien) 2004;146(10):1075–82 [discussion: 1082–3].
12. Smits M, Dippel DW, de Haan GG, et al. External validation of the Canadian CT Head Rule and the New Orleans Criteria for CT scanning in patients with minor head injury. JAMA 2005;294(12):1519–25.
13. Borg J, Holm L, Cassidy JD, et al. Diagnostic procedures in mild traumatic brain injury: results of the WHO Collaborating Centre Task Force on mild traumatic brain injury. J Rehabil Med 2004;43(Suppl):61–75.
14. af Geijerstam JL, Britton M. Mild head injury-mortality and complication rate: meta-analysis of findings in a systematic literature review. Acta Neurochir (Wien) 2003;145(10):843–50 [discussion: 850].
15. Teasdale GM, Murray G, Anderson E, et al. Risks of acute traumatic intracranial haematoma in children and adults: implications for managing head injuries. BMJ 1990;300(6721):363–7.
16. Hofman PA, Nelemans P, Kemerink GJ, et al. Value of radiological diagnosis of skull fracture in the management of mild head injury: meta-analysis. J Neurol Neurosurg Psychiatry 2000;68(4):416–22.
17. Lloyd DA, Carty H, Patterson M, et al. Predictive value of skull radiography for intracranial injury in children with blunt head injury. Lancet 1997;349(9055): 821–4.
18. Practice parameter: the management of concussion in sports (summary statement). Report of the Quality Standards Subcommittee. Neurology 1997;48(3):581–5.
19. Guskiewicz KM, Bruce SL, Cantu RC, et al. National Athletic Trainers' Association Position statement: management of sport-related concussion. J Athl Train 2004; 39(3):280–97.
20. Concussion (mild traumatic brain injury) and the team physician: a consensus statement. Med Sci Sports Exerc 2005;37(11):2012–6.
21. Ginde AA, Foianini A, Renner DM, et al. Availability and quality of computed tomography and magnetic resonance imaging equipment in U.S. emergency departments. Acad Emerg Med 2008;15(8):780–3.
22. Huda W, Vance A. Patient radiation doses from adult and pediatric CT. AJR Am J Roentgenol 2007;188(2):540–6.
23. Bushberg JT, Seibert JA, Leidholdt EM Jr, et al. The essential physics of medical imaging. 2nd edition. Philadelphia: Lippincott Williams & Wilkins; 2002.
24. McNitt-Gray MF. AAPM/RSNA Physics tutorial for residents: topics in CT. Radiation dose in CT. Radiographics 2002;22(6):1541–53.
25. Smith-Bindman R, Lipson J, Marcus R, et al. Radiation dose associated with common computed tomography examinations and the associated lifetime attributable risk of cancer. Arch Intern Med 2009;169(22):2078–86.

26. King MA, Kanal KM, Relyea-Chew A, et al. Radiation exposure from pediatric head CT: a bi-institutional study. Pediatr Radiol 2009;39(10):1059–65.
27. Board of Radiation Effects Research Division on Earth and Life Sciences National Research Council of the National Academies. Health risks from exposure to low levels of ionizing radiation: BEIR VII Phase 2. Washington, DC: National Academies Press; 2006.
28. Stiell IG, Wells GA, Vandemheen K, et al. The Canadian CT Head Rule for patients with minor head injury. Lancet 2001;357(9266):1391–6.
29. Pooley RA. AAPM/RSNA physics tutorial for residents: fundamental physics of MR imaging. Radiographics 2005;25(4):1087–99.
30. Ashwal S, Babikian T, Gardner-Nichols J, et al. Susceptibility-weighted imaging and proton magnetic resonance spectroscopy in assessment of outcome after pediatric traumatic brain injury. Arch Phys Med Rehabil 2006;87(12 Suppl 2): S50–8.
31. Orrison WW, Gentry LR, Stimac GK, et al. Blinded comparison of cranial CT and MR in closed head injury evaluation. AJNR Am J Neuroradiol 1994;15(2):351–6.
32. Gentry LR, Godersky JC, Thompson B, et al. Prospective comparative study of intermediate-field MR and CT in the evaluation of closed head trauma. AJR Am J Roentgenol 1988;150(3):673–82.
33. Lee H, Wintermark M, Gean AD, et al. Focal lesions in acute mild traumatic brain injury and neurocognitive outcome: CT versus 3T MRI. J Neurotrauma 2008; 25(9):1049–56.
34. Jordan BD, Zimmerman RD. Computed tomography and magnetic resonance imaging comparisons in boxers. JAMA 1990;263(12):1670–4.
35. af Geijerstam JL, Britton M. Mild head injury: reliability of early computed tomographic findings in triage for admission. Emerg Med J 2005;22(2):103–7.
36. Holbourn A. Mechanics of head injury. Lancet 1943;242(6267):438–41.
37. Graham DI, Adams JH, Nicoll JA, et al. The nature, distribution and causes of traumatic brain injury. Brain Pathol 1995;5(4):397–406.
38. Barkhoudarian G, Hovda DA, Giza CC. The molecular pathophysiology of concussive brain injury. Clin Sports Med 2011;30(1):33–48, vii–iii.
39. Li XY, Feng DF. Diffuse axonal injury: novel insights into detection and treatment. J Clin Neurosci 2009;16(5):614–9.
40. Paterakis K, Karantanas AH, Komnos A, et al. Outcome of patients with diffuse axonal injury: the significance and prognostic value of MRI in the acute phase. J Trauma 2000;49(6):1071–5.
41. Marquez de la Plata C, Ardelean A, Koovakkattu D, et al. Magnetic resonance imaging of diffuse axonal injury: quantitative assessment of white matter lesion volume. J Neurotrauma 2007;24(4):591–8.
42. Spain A, Daumas S, Lifshitz J, et al. Mild fluid percussion injury in mice produces evolving selective axonal pathology and cognitive deficits relevant to human brain injury. J Neurotrauma 2010;27(8):1429–38.
43. Yeo RA, Phillips JP, Jung RE, et al. Magnetic resonance spectroscopy detects brain injury and predicts cognitive functioning in children with brain injuries. J Neurotrauma 2006;23(10):1427–35.
44. Henry LC, Tremblay S, Boulanger Y, et al. Neurometabolic changes in the acute phase after sports concussions correlate with symptom severity. J Neurotrauma 2010;27(1):65–76.
45. Vagnozzi R, Signoretti S, Tavazzi B, et al. Temporal window of metabolic brain vulnerability to concussion: a pilot 1H-magnetic resonance spectroscopic study in concussed athletes—part III. Neurosurgery 2008;62(6):1286–95 [discussion: 1295–6].

46. Sinson G, Bagley LJ, Cecil KM, et al. Magnetization transfer imaging and proton MR spectroscopy in the evaluation of axonal injury: correlation with clinical outcome after traumatic brain injury. AJNR Am J Neuroradiol 2001;22(1):143–51.

47. Cecil KM, Hills EC, Sandel ME, et al. Proton magnetic resonance spectroscopy for detection of axonal injury in the splenium of the corpus callosum of brain-injured patients. J Neurosurg 1998;88(5):795–801.

48. Govindaraju V, Gauger GE, Manley GT, et al. Volumetric proton spectroscopic imaging of mild traumatic brain injury. AJNR Am J Neuroradiol 2004;25(5):730–7.

49. Garnett MR, Corkill RG, Blamire AM, et al. Altered cellular metabolism following traumatic brain injury: a magnetic resonance spectroscopy study. J Neurotrauma 2001;18(3):231–40.

50. Le Bihan D, Mangin JF, Poupon C, et al. Diffusion tensor imaging: concepts and applications. J Magn Reson Imaging 2001;13(4):534–46.

51. Johansen-Berg H, Rushworth MF. Using diffusion imaging to study human connectional anatomy. Annu Rev Neurosci 2009;32:75–94.

52. Cubon VA, Putukian M, Boyer C, et al. A diffusion tensor imaging study on the white matter skeleton in individuals with sports-related concussion. J Neurotrauma 2011; 28(2):189–201.

53. Smits M, Houston GC, Dippel DW, et al. Microstructural brain injury in post-concussion syndrome after minor head injury. Neuroradiology 2011;53(8): 553–63.

54. Niogi SN, Mukherjee P, Ghajar J, et al. Extent of microstructural white matter injury in postconcussive syndrome correlates with impaired cognitive reaction time: a 3T diffusion tensor imaging study of mild traumatic brain injury. AJNR Am J Neuroradiol 2008;29(5):967–73.

55. Lipton ML, Gellella E, Lo C, et al. Multifocal white matter ultrastructural abnormalities in mild traumatic brain injury with cognitive disability: a voxel-wise analysis of diffusion tensor imaging. J Neurotrauma 2008;25(11):1335–42.

56. Mayer AR, Ling J, Mannell MV, et al. A prospective diffusion tensor imaging study in mild traumatic brain injury. Neurology 2010;74(8):643–50.

57. Wilde EA, McCauley SR, Hunter JV, et al. Diffusion tensor imaging of acute mild traumatic brain injury in adolescents. Neurology 2008;70(12):948–55.

58. Ptito A, Chen JK, Johnston KM. Contributions of functional magnetic resonance imaging (fMRI) to sport concussion evaluation. NeuroRehabilitation 2007;22(3): 217–27.

59. Chen JK, Johnston KM, Petrides M, et al. Recovery from mild head injury in sports: evidence from serial functional magnetic resonance imaging studies in male athletes. Clin J Sport Med 2008;18(3):241–7.

60. Chen JK, Johnston KM, Frey S, et al. Functional abnormalities in symptomatic concussed athletes: an fMRI study. Neuroimage 2004;22(1):68–82.

61. Jantzen KJ, Anderson B, Steinberg FL, et al. A prospective functional MR imaging study of mild traumatic brain injury in college football players. AJNR Am J Neuroradiol 2004;25(5):738–45.

62. Lovell MR, Pardini JE, Welling J, et al. Functional brain abnormalities are related to clinical recovery and time to return-to-play in athletes. Neurosurgery 2007; 61(2):352–9 [discussion: 359–60].

63. McAllister TW, Sparling MB, Flashman LA, et al. Differential working memory load effects after mild traumatic brain injury. Neuroimage 2001;14(5):1004–12.

64. Chen SH, Kareken DA, Fastenau PS, et al. A study of persistent post-concussion symptoms in mild head trauma using positron emission tomography. J Neurol Neurosurg Psychiatry 2003;74(3):326–32.

65. Umile EM, Sandel ME, Alavi A, et al. Dynamic imaging in mild traumatic brain injury: support for the theory of medial temporal vulnerability. Arch Phys Med Rehabil 2002;83(11):1506–13.

66. Gross H, Kling A, Henry G, et al. Local cerebral glucose metabolism in patients with long-term behavioral and cognitive deficits following mild traumatic brain injury. J Neuropsychiatry Clin Neurosci 1996;8(3):324–34.

67. Ruff RM, Crouch JA, Troster AI, et al. Selected cases of poor outcome following a minor brain trauma: comparing neuropsychological and positron emission tomography assessment. Brain Inj 1994;8(4):297–308.

68. Abu-Judeh HH, Parker R, Singh M, et al. SPET brain perfusion imaging in mild traumatic brain injury without loss of consciousness and normal computed tomography. Nucl Med Commun 1999;20(6):505–10.

69. Bonne O, Gilboa A, Louzoun Y, et al. Cerebral blood flow in chronic symptomatic mild traumatic brain injury. Psychiatry Res 2003;124(3):141–52.

Use of Neuropsychological Evaluations

David B. Coppel, PhD[a,b,*]

KEYWORDS

• Neuropsychology • Sports concussion • Evaluation
• Brain dysfunction

Neuropsychology is an applied science that is concerned with the behavioral expression of brain dysfunction. Although neurology and neurosurgery are focused primarily on the brain and its structural and nervous system integrity and functions, clinical neuropsychology focuses primarily on the mind, or how the brain interacts with the world. These cognitive, or neurocognitive, functions of the brain involve receptive and expressive functions, attention and concentration, and information processing, and the integrative functions of learning and memory and problem solving. Neurocognitive skills relate to how individuals track or select and acquire information, store and retrieve information, organize information for problem solving, and express or communicate. Emotions, and emotional functioning, have a bidirectional relationship with neurocognition, in that brain-based difficulties can cause emotional disturbance and emotional status can affect cognitive functioning.

Mild head injury or concussion is often characterized by cognitive symptoms in the form of attention or concentration problems, slowed processing, and/or memory difficulties. An individual may display minimal symptoms, and usually has a normal neurologic examination, but still has subtle changes in functioning; these differences from preinjury functioning may be observed by others and/or felt by the individual ("I don't feel right" or "I don't feel like myself"). In addition to the common physically based symptoms of sports concussions, such as headache, dizziness, balance problems, or sleep disturbance, subtle cognitive symptoms may be present, including reduced planning and ability to switch mental set, impaired memory and learning, reduced attention and ability to process information, and slowed reaction times and increased variability in response.[1] The sports culture/context, and its influence on minimization of self-reported symptoms,[2] created a need to evaluate cognitive

[a] Department of Neurosurgery, Harborview Medical Center, Box 359766, 325 Ninth Avenue, Seattle, WA 98104-2499, USA
[b] Seattle Sports Concussion Program, Box 359721, 325 Ninth Avenue, Seattle, WA 98104, USA
* Department of Neurosurgery, Harborview Medical Center, Box 359766, 325 Ninth Avenue, Seattle, WA 98104-2499.
E-mail address: dcoppel@uw.edu

Phys Med Rehabil Clin N Am 22 (2011) 653–664
doi:10.1016/j.pmr.2011.08.006
1047-9651/11/$ – see front matter © 2011 Elsevier Inc. All rights reserved.

functioning beyond the basic cognitive tests contained in a mental status examination or the reliance on self-reported cognitive functioning.[3] Cognitive symptoms of concussion can persist beyond the resolution of major physical symptoms,[3–5] and emotional symptoms from concussion can emerge as primary symptoms of head injury (eg, emotional lability or irritability) and/or reactive or secondary responses to symptoms or circumstances (eg, depression, discouragement or frustration with physical activity restriction, or interpersonal interaction changes).[6,7] Increased risk of depression for those with mild traumatic brain injury has been found.[8] This increased risk for depression extends to concussed athletes and has incorporated neuroimaging research; Chen and colleagues[9] found that athletes with concussion with depressive symptoms showed neuroimaging patterns of activation and deactivation consistent with those found in clinical depression (ie, reduced activation in dorsolateral prefrontal cortex and striatum and attenuated deactivation in medial frontal and temporal regions).

EMERGENCE OF SPORTS NEUROPSYCHOLOGY

The role of neuropsychology in a clinical setting can be to evaluate neurocognitive areas of functioning and relate the pattern of results to events (eg, traumatic brain injury), brain disease, and/or current level of functioning. These results can provide significant input to management and treatment of conditions. Neuropsychological assessments provide performance-based data (in contrast with self-report) that can document the level or degree of relative deficits and delineate areas of relative strength. Neuropsychology has played an important role in the understanding and evaluation of traumatic brain injury and its impact on adaptive functioning for many decades.[10,11] The role of neuropsychology in mild traumatic brain injuries in sports, most often referred to as sports concussions, has created a growing field referred to as sports neuropsychology.[12–15]

The application of neuropsychological approaches to sports concussions developed largely from the work of Barth and colleagues[16,17] and the development of the Sports as a Laboratory Assessment Model (SLAM), which was oriented to using information from sports-related concussion to help inform the evaluation of mild head injury in the general population. In most clinical settings, clinical neuropsychological evaluations are in response to a brain trauma event and preinjury data are not available. Barth and colleagues[16,17] used the sports environment and the opportunity to assess athletes before injury, thus creating the basis for the current approach to sports concussion that involves baseline testing and follow-up. The neuropsychological test batteries that have evolved from the early work of Barth and colleagues[16,17] have been developed to evaluate areas of neurocognitive functioning most often affected by mild brain injury/concussion; these areas include attention/concentration; new learning; speeded problem solving, processing speed, and short-term memory; visual tracking; and balance testing, and these areas have been included in some evaluation approaches. Some neurocognitive test batteries add tests that assess areas that are not typically negatively affected by mild head injury and may serve as preinjury performance level estimates.

Comprehensive neuropsychological evaluations generally include a detailed clinical interview that not only explores the history of the present illness/injury but also history and background of the individual (social, educational, occupational, medical histories), review of available records, and neuropsychological testing to evaluate areas of cognitive functioning including intellectual functions, academic skills, attention and concentration, processing speed, learning, memory, psychomotor functions, and emotional functioning. This evaluation process provides an opportunity to observe individuals in their problem-solving efforts and make neurobehavioral observations. The neuro-psychological report can describe the pattern and ranges of performance, and determine whether the pattern is consistent with the history of present illness and current symptoms. The neuropsychologist integrates the history, neurocognitive findings, medical data, and psychosocial-emotional factors and provides impressions regarding the individual's current status, and may make recommendations for treatment planning.

In contrast with comprehensive clinical neuropsychological evaluations, sports concussion evaluations have generally focused on areas of functioning most often affected by concussion and are structured as neurocognitive screenings; having a pre-injury or baseline performance level for comparison has emerged as the predominant paradigm. These evaluations are often administered sequentially (serial testing) to track neurocognitive status through the recovery phase; thus, alternate or multiple forms of tests are important to minimize the confounding of neurocognitive improvement and improvement caused by practice (or prior exposure) effects. Computerized neurocognitive testing for sports-related concussion[18] solves the problem of alternate equivalent forms by generating multiple versions of subtests. However, although the content changes, the procedural practice effect (prior exposure to procedures and how the subtest works) remains.

Roles of Neuropsychological Evaluations in Sports Concussion

The roles of neuropsychological, or neurocognitive, evaluations in sports concussion have been seen in various ways, often seemingly dependent on the makeup of the expert group, as the sports concussion field has developed with time. The initial Concussion in Sports Group consensus statement[19] promoted neuropsychological assessment as an important part of the evaluation of concussion protocol. This statement was followed by the second consensus statement, which described neuropsychological testing as being useful and important in the evaluation and management of complex concussions (which are contrasted with simple concussions, and relate to prolonged or slow recovery), and acknowledged the value of baseline and serial testing.[20] The most recent consensus group statement[21] recognized neuropsychological assessment as a useful tool in return-to-play decisions, and baseline testing, if possible, was again recommended. It was emphasized that neuropsychological assessment should not be seen as the "sole basis of management decisions, rather it should be seen as an aid to the clinical decision-making process in conjunction with a range of clinical domains and investigational results." The essential aspect of this position regarding neuropsychological assessment is that it is but 1 data point among many that should be considered in concussion evaluation and management; this multidisciplinary approach, if possible, allows for the most comprehensive evaluation and management input for athletes as they recover.

The value of neuropsychological testing has been generally established in assessing or documenting cognitive problems emerging from sports-related concussion.[3,22–27] Assessment strategies have varied from the traditional paper-and-pencil tests, to test batteries, to multiple options for computerized neurocognitive testing. Neurocognitive tasks are included in many of the brief sideline evaluations (eg, Standardized Assessment of Concussion [SAC[28,29]]), and assess orientation, auditory memory (immediate and delayed), concentration (digit span), and sequencing (months backward). These brief sideline evaluations provide a general view of functions and are not usually able to detect subtle changes in neurocognitive function emerging from concussion[30]; further, the sideline evaluators may not have a baseline performance level with which to compare an athlete's postinjury performance level for memory or auditory attention tasks (eg, digit span). The sideline evaluation for concussion usually assesses symptoms and general responsiveness, postural stability and coordination, and the aforementioned brief cognitive functions, which usually provide current status information that informs clinical management decisions.

The use of neuropsychological testing for evaluation and management of sport-related concussion makes intuitive sense because it provides a measurement, or quantification, of cognitive function and emerges from a long history of application in brain injury evaluation. The inclusion of baseline testing in the testing protocol, as initially used by Barth and colleagues[17] and now with other systems, provides each athlete with a nonconcussed comparison point. Evaluation of the changes in performance, and the pattern of changes for the different tests are the crucial analyses. Recognizing a decline as being significantly different (not occurring by chance or normal variability) and reliable measurement are the major challenges for the evaluator.[31] The reliability, validity, sensitivity, and clinical usefulness of neuropsychological testing has been scrutinized and found by some to have not met criteria for clinical use.[30,32] However, other research has provided some reliability and validity data that support neurocognitive testing[33,34]; the usage of reliable change indices is helpful in interpretation of the test data.[35] Despite the ongoing need for more research regarding reliability and validity of measures with athlete populations,[36] the use of neuropsychological or neurocognitive testing (within the baseline comparison protocol) has expanded and is a useful, important, and, in some contexts, a recommended or mandated aspect of concussion management.

Computer-Based Neurocognitive Testing

The development of computer-administered tests of cognitive functions grew out of the need to evaluate large numbers of athletes quickly and cost-efficiently; in contrast, traditional neuropsychological assessment requires more time and labor in terms of using a neuropsychologist.[37–40] Computerized assessment also provides more exact measurement of reaction time and processing speed, both of which are important aspects in concussion-related performance changes. Lovell[37] further suggested that the traditional approaches (noncomputer) limited the widespread use of neuropsychological assessment, especially at and below high school levels. Computer-based approaches have been used in youth athlete groups at all competitive ranges; however, hopes for expansion of involvement of neuropsychologists in sport settings have yet to be fulfilled. The various computerized neurocognitive assessment programs provide neurocognitive test data (scores or composite scores) that are subsequently interpreted for purposes of treatment planning and/or return-to-play decisions.

Although the administration of these computerized neurocognitive tests can be completed by an athletic trainer or someone trained in the administration and setup, it is the interpretation of the neurocognitive test data that has been variable. Echemendia and colleagues[41] opine that, although baseline testing can be conducted by technicians with the supervision or guidance of a neuropsychologist, "post-injury assessment requires advanced neuropsychological expertise that is best provided by a clinical neuropsychologist." They further suggest that interpretation responsibility may be seen in a medicolegal context and scope-of-practice issues can be raised. Despite the availability of hours of workshop training for nonneuropsychologists, the interpretation of computer-based neurocognitive tests is best completed by a trained, qualified neuropsychologist.

The complex factors that may affect neuropsychological test performance, specified by Collie and colleagues,[39] include clinical (concussion/head injury, depression/anxiety/mood state, fatigue, use of drugs and alcohol, other medical or psychological conditions), methodological (testing situation, practice or learning effects, administrator expertise), test related (types of cognition assessed, availability of alternative forms, test reliability and/or repeatability, regression to the mean), statistical (metric properties, outcome variables such as reaction time and accuracy, statistical analysis used), and other (chance, random variability). It is the integration of these clinical and nonclinical factors with the individual test results that is the particular purview of neuropsychologists. Computerized programs that produce statistically determined results regarding return to baseline levels/ranges, or not returned to baseline, provide important information, but often provide an oversimplification of the complex system of cognitive functioning and the influence of other factors.

By virtue of their training and skill sets, neuropsychologists can provide "unique expertise in the assessment of cognitive functioning and post-injury neurocognitive and psychological assessment."[42] Moser and colleagues[27] describe clinical neuropsychologists as uniquely qualified to translate test data into recommendations for clinical management; neuropsychological evaluation is recommended for use in the diagnosis, treatment, and management of sports-related concussion at all levels of play. Carr and Shunk[43] detail training and qualifications of a sport neuropsychologist, suggesting that neuropsychologists should have additional training and specialization in the application of their clinical skills in the sports environment and with an athlete population. They emphasize the ethical responsibility of the psychologist to seek training to gain competency in this newly developing area.

The use of baseline testing has emerged as a crucial part of concussion management protocols, but the usefulness of this baseline model has been questioned[44]; psychometric and methodological issues are not at a level that justifies the implementation of a baseline testing system. Specifically, it is claimed that there are no studies showing that baseline testing reduces the duration of postconcussive symptoms, or the likelihood of repeat concussion, or the severity of symptoms or neurocognitive dysfunction after a second concussion, so the clinical use for return-to-play decisions is premature.[42] Although these are important points regarding neurocognitive testing and its validity and sensitivity, the role for neurocognitive testing as one of many tools in clinical management and return-to-play decisions may not be fully appreciated. In addition to questions regarding the baseline model, some practitioners have believed that results from computerized testing do not add value beyond their own clinically informed decisions regarding return to play. Symptomatic athletes are generally not ready for return to play, regardless of their neurocognitive test results, so its added value for the return decision may be low; asymptomatic athletes (self-report) may or may not be ready for return to play and having some neurocognitive data describing their level of function (relative to a nonconcussed level) can be a helpful adjunct in return-to-play or management decisions. Poor, or below baseline, neurocognitive testing results, within the context of an asymptomatic report, at the least, will hopefully trigger additional consideration by the practitioner, especially if the athlete is also involved in school/academic activities. In some cases, the measurement, description, and tracking of the relative cognitive strengths and weaknesses and improvement for athletes during recovery can provide a helpful and adaptive perspective. Neurocognitive testing did show some degree of value-added benefits beyond self-report of symptoms,[3,45] and may be helpful to the practitioner (especially with the involvement of a neuropsychologist) in detecting some of the subtle cognitive changes associated with concussion/mild traumatic brain injury that may not be within their specialty.

Randolph[46] and others, in their discussions regarding baseline testing issues, suggest that baseline testing does not modify serious risks associated with sport-related concussion, noting that there "is no way that baseline testing could prevent a prolonged or atypical recovery, although in theory, baseline testing could help track recovery (presuming the tests were sufficiently reliable)." Although the evidence for baseline testing being able to modify risk or prevent serious outcomes in sports-related concussion is not available, the use of neuropsychological or neurocognitive testing to evaluate ongoing, prolonged, or atypical recovery is believed to be professionally prudent, with neuropsychologists being trained to integrate these data with the athlete's history and potential risk factors.

Within a baseline neurocognitive testing and follow-up to concussion approach, the follow-up measures of functioning are of greatest use with a valid baseline comparison measure. Some athletes have been known to intentionally perform poorly on baseline to create a low comparison point to evaluate change on postconcussion follow-up; thus, any concussion-related cognitive decline may still be in their baseline range and suggest no cognitive residuals. Most athletes seem generally motivated to make a good effort at follow-up (which they perceive may help them be cleared to play), but some athletes have other issues or factors that affect their effort and performance. They may believe that they have to continue to display difficulties to support their injury, or they may be looking for an honorable or acceptable reason (eg, continuing to show ongoing symptoms) to discontinue participation, or other psychosocial factors may be involved. In some cases, youth athletes are able to access classroom or homework accommodations in school as long as they are experiencing concussion-related symptoms, which may relate to poor effort and performance on baseline or follow-up testing. Studies regarding baseline testing have revealed that psychological distress symptoms at the time of testing accounted for a significant amount of the baseline neurocognitive performance. This finding suggests the need for screening for psychological symptoms at baseline and follow-up concussion evaluations.[47,48] Although it is intuitive to think of athletes being highly motivated individuals, their performances on neurocognitive testing can reflect variable effort; although they may display good effort on follow-up because it could affect return-to-play decisions, their baseline performances are often low and reflective of poor effort.[49] Hunt and colleagues[49] found that 11% of the high school athletes exerted poor effort and produced lowered or invalid neurocognitive performance on baseline testing, which could affect subsequent follow-up interpretation; the inclusion of an effort measure in a concussion assessment battery is recommended. For youth athletes, more frequent baseline testing is indicated, because the brain continues to develop and cognitively mature in adolescence. Some computer-based concussion programs recommend a new baseline yearly or every 2 years in youth athletes.

Although computerized baseline and follow-up neurocognitive testing has provided a response to the issues of the high number of athletes to be tested, relative cost and time, and alternate test forms, the computer-based approach has significant limitations regarding the information obtained. Specifically, the computer-based approach provides no information regarding auditory processing or verbal-auditory memory, because it is all visually presented; information regarding auditory processing or auditory attention can be particularly important for youth athletes and the impact on school or classroom performance and functioning. The computer-based evaluations provide data based on visual recognition memory, not recall memory; this is of note because recognition memory is more likely to be preserved in mild traumatic brain injury and recall memory more likely to be affected. Recognition memory tasks involve identifying stimuli from presented choices, recall memory tasks involve generating the stimuli from memory. In contrast with traditional face-to-face testing, computerized testing provides no neurobehavioral observational data regarding problem-solving efforts, distractibility, expressive or receptive language, motor skills, or emotional responses.

The hybrid model described by Echemendia[50] involves the combination of computer and traditional face-to-face testing. In this way, the important reaction time data and general cognitive efficiency (speed vs accuracy) is used from the computerized testing, and the memory, problem-solving, and neurobehavioral observations can be used from the face-to-face testing. This hybrid approach may be particularly useful with athletes with certain risk factors, such as preexisting learning disabilities or attention-deficit/hyperactivity disorder, history of migraine headache, prior brain/head trauma, illnesses or diseases that may have compromised neurocognitive functioning, and psychiatric/psychological disorders. The expanded battery of neurocognitive tests may give the practitioner additional information to use in the description of the athlete's current status and any return-to-play decision or treatment planning.

Pediatric and Adolescent Sport Concussion Management

Sport concussion issues specific to pediatric and adolescent athlete populations center on concussion management issues for these athletes being distinct from adult athletes and call for a more conservative approach.[51–54] Children are believed to have increased susceptibility to concussion and potentially worse neuropsychological outcomes based on their neurodevelopmental status, including incomplete myelination of brain axons, greater head/body ratio, and thinner cranial bones.[55,56] With the primary research emphasis being on college or professional athlete concussions and concussion management, Kirkwood and colleagues[57] describe pediatric sport-related concussed athletes as "an oft-neglected population." As the epidemiology of postconcussion symptoms is researched and described,[58] youth sport concussion is becoming seen as a growing health concern.[59] An 11-year prospective study of high school concussion incidence[60] found that the rate increased across all 12 sports studied, with the concussion rate increasing 4.2-fold, reflecting a 15.5% annual increase.

Most practitioners dealing with sports-related concussion or mild traumatic brain injury acknowledge that having some form of neurocognitive or neuropsychological test data to supplement other medical, physiologic, or historical data is helpful in the clinical management of these athletes. Neurocognitive test data are generally not believed to be a stand-alone measure for return-to-play decisions, but are among several data points to be considered. Similarly, patient self-report of the absence of postconcussion symptoms or a normal balance performance should not solely be relied on to determine return-to-play status. In many concussion management programs, a multidisciplinary or interdisciplinary team approach is used. Uniquely, neuropsychologists can provide the team, program, or physician managing youth concussions with (1) age-normed data regarding neurocognitive functioning, (2) recommendations regarding potentially important issues related to academic functioning, and (3) assessment of social-emotional functioning or psychosocial issues that have affected functioning levels. In addition, neuropsychologists can interface, if needed, with parents and school regarding ongoing concussion issues. The neuropsychological evaluation integrates the physical, cognitive, and emotional aspects of sports-related concussions, and considers alternative explanations and factors symptoms persist.

SUMMARY

Neuropsychological testing has been used for decades in the evaluation of mild traumatic brain injury and the application of this area to sports concussion has helped to develop sports neuropsychology. These neuropsychological or neurocognitive test results provide information regarding the cognitive status (and emotional status, in some cases) of the concussed athlete. The availability of preinjury or baseline data regarding an athlete's level of cognitive functioning can provide an important marker for comparison with postinjury performance levels. Although these before-and-after injury comparisons may be influenced by many noninjury factors, these results can provide some normative measurement of cognition, and some indication of the impact of the concussion injury on cognitive functioning. The development and availability of computerized testing platforms has allowed the widespread application of the baseline and follow-up testing model at all levels of athletic involvement, and provide a more precise measurement of reaction time and processing speed. However, the ease and convenience of computerized testing has sacrificed some important aspects of neurocognitive or neuropsychological testing, such as neurobehavioral observations, auditory processing performance, recall memory measurement, and assessment of psychosocial and emotional factors. In addition, computerized testing has created (and advertised/marketed) the oversimplification of neurocognitive status assessment down to statistical change assessment (similar to blood test results), and suggests to some practitioners that cognitive issues have been addressed. In many instances, there are more questions to be asked and more cognitive data to be obtained, and, in particular, more factors to be considered. The hybrid model, which involves a combination of computerized assessment and a more expanded battery of tests, seems to be a prudent approach to better understanding the often complex nature of the cognitive impact of sports concussion in youth athletes. This approach may be especially important for athletes with general risk factors (for prolonged recovery) and other potential modifiers or influencers on the cognitive performance data; some of these factors include history of learning disabilities, attention deficit disorder, psychiatric history, history of migraine or other headache conditions, significant psychological or psychosocial issues, sleep disorders, prior brain trauma (sports related and non–sports related), ongoing medical conditions and metabolism issues, and potential medication effects.

Neuropsychological or neurocognitive testing can provide the sport medicine practitioner(s) or team caring for athletes with important information regarding cognitive residual functioning after concussion, which is one aspect of the decision for an athlete to return to play, but is perhaps the most far reaching for youth athletes. These test results reflect the brain's efficiency and general capacity for processing and cognition following a concussion and during the course of recovery. As indicated previously, these results are best interpreted and communicated (to the sports medicine practitioner and, in some cases, to the athlete and family) by a qualified neuropsychologist.

As the use of computerized neuropsychological testing for sports-related concussion management continues to expand, access to neuropsychological consultation becomes a crucial need. Although the availability of neuropsychologists to directly evaluate individual athletes may be limited or nonexistent in some areas, neuropsychologists may have greater availability to provide consultation to team physicians, athletic trainers, or other sports medicine providers regarding test results of concussed athletes. For example, as part of the Seattle Sports Concussion Program, neuropsychologists review all computerized neuropsychological test data from concussion follow-ups in participating high schools in the Seattle School District and other school districts and provide consultation regarding the results to athletic trainers and sports medicine providers. This consultation begins with obtaining some basic background information regarding the athlete and the injury, and continues with feedback to the athletic trainer regarding the test data and their meaning for the individual athlete, and directed follow-up questions regarding the athlete, symptoms, and observed behavior. These exchanges provide for a more effective interpretation (and understanding) of follow-up test data for the individual athlete, which contributes to return-to-play decisions and initiation of return-to-play protocols. The neuropsychologist may also indicate the need for more expanded testing and other recommendations or referrals. Developing a consultative relationship with a neuropsychologist, even for remote consultation, allows a program to make best use of computerized testing and provide guidance with the test data, given their limitations. The development and use of telemedicine or telehealth systems for this consultative purpose in rural or underserved regions is another approach to potentially providing the best available evaluation and management to more concussed athletes.

Neuropsychology will continue to scrutinize the tests and testing approaches for validity, reliability, and related issues in these sports concussion populations, and research the influences of risk factors on cognitive performance and recovery in sports concussion. It is hoped that these efforts will help provide information regarding cognitive and emotional effects of sports concussion and lead toward development of even more effective and meaningful measures and resources for youth athletes.

REFERENCES

1. McCrory P, Makdissi M, Davis G, et al. Value of neuropsychological testing after head injuries in football. Br J Sports Med 2005;39(Suppl 1):i58–63.
2. McCrea M, Hammeke T, Olsen G, et al. Unreported concussion in high school football players: implications for prevention. Clin J Sport Med 2004;14:13–7.
3. Van Kampen D, Lovell M, Pardini J, et al. The "value added" of neurocognitive testing after sports-related concussion. Am J Sports Med 2006;34(10):1630–5.
4. Collins M, Field M, Lovell M, et al. Relationship between postconcussion headache and neuropsychological test performance in high school athletes. Am J Sports Med 2003;31(2):168–73.
5. Broglio S, Macciocchi S, Ferrara M. Neurocognitive performance of concussed athletes when symptom free. J Athl Train 2007;42(4):504–8.
6. Mainwaring L. Short-term and extended emotional correlates of concussion. In: Webbe F, editor. The handbook of sport neuropsychology. New York (NY): Springer; 2010. p. 251–73.
7. Mainwaring L, Bisschop S, Green R, et al. Emotional reactions of varsity athletes to sport-related concussion. J Sport Exerc Psychol 2004;26:119–35.
8. Fann J, Burington B, Leonetti A, et al. Psychiatric illness following traumatic brain injury in adult health maintenance organization population. Arch Gen Psychiatry 2004;61:53–61.
9. Chen J, Johnston K, Petrides M, et al. Neural substrates of symptoms of depression following concussion in male athletes with persisting postconcussion symptoms. Arch Gen Psychiatry 2008;65(1):81–9.
10. Levin HS, Eisenberg HM, Benton AL, editors. Mild head injury. New York (NY): Oxford University Press; 1989.
11. Dikman S, McLean A, Temkin N. Neuropsychological and psychosocial consequences of minor head injury. J Neurol Neurosurg Psychiatr 1986;49:1227–32.
12. Barth JT, Broshek DK, Freeman JR. A new frontier for neuropsychology. In: Echemendia R, editor. Sports neuropsychology: assessment and management of traumatic brain injury. New York (NY): Guilford Press; 2006.
13. Webbe FM, editor. The handbook of sport neuropsychology. New York (NY): Springer; 2010.
14. Bailes JE, Lovell MR, Maroon JC, editors. Sport related concussion. St Louis (MO): Quality Medical Publishing; 1999.

15. Echemendia RJ, Julian LJ. Mild traumatic brain injury in sports: neuropsychology's contribution to a developing field. Neuropsychol Rev 2001;11:69–88.
16. Barth J, Harvey D, Freeman J, et al. Sport as a laboratory assessment model. In: Webbe F, editor. The handbook of sport neuropsychology. New York (NY): Springer; 2010. p. 75–89.
17. Barth J, Alves W, Ryan T, et al. Mild head injury in sports: neuropsychological sequelae and recovery of function. In: Levin H, Eisenberg H, Benton A, editors. Mild head injury. New York (NY): Oxford University Press; 1989. p. 257–75.
18. Schatz P, Zillmer E. Computer-based assessment of sports-related concussion. Appl Neuropsychol 2003;10(1):42–7.
19. Aubry M, Cantu R, Dvorak J, et al. Summary and agreement statement of 1st International symposium in concussion in sport, Vienna. Clin J Sport Med 2002; 12:6–11.
20. McCrory P, Johnston K, Meeuwise W, et al. Summary and agreement statement of the 2nd International conference on concussion in sport, Prague. Br J Sports Med 2005;29:196–204.
21. McCrory P, Meeuwise W, Johnston K, et al. Consensus statement on concussion in sport-The 3rd International conference on concussion in sport, Zurich, November 2008. J Clin Neurosci 2009;16(6):755–63.
22. Iverson G. Evidenced-based neuropsychological assessment in sport-related concussion. In: Webbe F, editor. The handbook of sport neuropsychology. New York (NY): Springer; 2010. p. 131–53.
23. Belanger H, Vanderploeg R. The neuropsychological impact of sport-related concussion: a meta-analysis. J Int Neuropsychol Soc 2005;11(4):345–57.
24. Broglio S, Macciocchi S, Ferrara M. Sensitivity of the concussion assessment battery. Neurosurgery 2007;60(6):1050–7.
25. Collins M, Grindel S, Lovell M, et al. Relationship between concussion and neuropsychological performance in college football players. JAMA 1999;282(10):964–70.
26. Echemendia R, Putukian M, Mackin R, et al. Neuropsychological test performance prior to and following sports-related mild traumatic brain injury. Clin J Sport Med 2001;11(1):23–31.
27. Moser R, Iverson G, Echemendia R, et al. Neuropsychological evaluation in the diagnosis and management of sports-related concussion. Arch Clin Neuropsychol 2007;22(8):909–16.
28. Barr W. Assessing mild traumatic brain injury on the sideline. In: Echemendia R, editor. Sports neuropsychology. New York (NY): Guilford Press; 2006. p. 87–109.
29. McCrea M, Kelly JP, Randolph C. Standardized assessment of concussion (SAC): on-site mental status evaluation of the athlete. J Head Trauma Rehabil 1998;13:27–35.
30. Randolph C, McCrea M, Barr W. Is Neuropsychological testing useful in the management of sport-related concussion? J Athl Train 2005;40(3):139–52.
31. Hinton-Bayre A, Geffen G, Geffen L, et al. Concussion in contact sports: reliable change indices of impairment and recovery. J Clin Exp Neuropsychol 1999;21(1): 70–86.
32. Grindel S. The use, abuse, and future of neuropsychologic testing in mild traumatic brain injury. Curr Sports Med Rep 2006;5:9–14.
33. Iverson G, Lovell M, Collins M. Validity of ImPACT for measuring the effects of sports-related concussion. Arch Clin Neuropsychol 2002;17(8):770.
34. Iverson G, Lovell M, Collins M. Validity of ImPACT for measuring processing speed following sports-related concussion. J Clin Exp Neuropsychol 2005; 27(6):683–9.

35. Iverson G, Lovell M, Collins M. Interpreting change on ImPACT following sports-related concussion. Clin Neuropsychol 2003;17(4):460–7.
36. Ellemberg D, Henry L, Macciocchi S, et al. Advances in sport concussion: from behavioral to brain injury measures. J Neurotrauma 2009;26:2365–82.
37. Lovell M. The ImPACT neuropsychological test battery. In: Echemendia R, editor. Sports neuropsychology. New York (NY): Guilford Press; 2006. p. 193–215.
38. Kaushik T, Erlanger D. The Headminder Concussion Resolution Index. In: Echemendia R, editor. Sports neuropsychology. New York (NY): Guilford Press; 2006. p. 216–39.
39. Collie A, Maruff P, Darby D, et al. CogSport. In: Echemendia R, editor. sports neuropsychology. New York (NY): Guilford Press; 2006. p. 240–62.
40. Bleiberg J, Cernich A, Reeves D. Sports concussion application of the automated neuropsychological assessment metrics sports medicine battery. In: Echemendia R, editor. Sports neuropsychology. New York (NY): Guilford Press; 2006. p. 263–83.
41. Echemendia RJ, Herring S, Bailes J. Who should conduct and interpret the neuropsychological assessment in sports-related concussion? Br J Sports Med 2009; 43(Suppl 1):i32–5.
42. Randolph C, Kirkwood M. What are the real risks of sport-related concussion and are they modifiable. J Int Neuropsychol Soc 2009;15(4):512–20.
43. Carr C, Shunk A. Qualifications and training of the sport neuropsychologist. In: Webbe F, editor. The handbook of sports neuropsychology. New York (NY): Springer; 2010. p. 17–34.
44. Kirkwood M, Randolph C, Yeates K. Returning pediatric athletes to play after concussion: the evidence (or lack thereof) behind baseline neuropsychological testing. Acta Paediatr 2009;98(9):1409–11.
45. Makdissi M, Darby D, Maruff P, et al. Natural history of concussion in sports: markers of severity and implications for management. Am J Sports Med 2010; 38:464–71.
46. Randolph C. Baseline neuropsychological testing in managing sport-related concussion: does it modify risk? Curr Sports Med Rep 2011;10(1):21–6.
47. Bailey C, Samples H, Broshek D, et al. The relationship between psychological distress and baseline sports-related concussion testing. Clin J Sport Med 2010;20(4):272–7.
48. Kirkwood M, Kirk J, Blaha R, et al. Non-credible effort during pediatric neuropsychological exam: a case series and literature review. Child Neuropsychology 2010;16:604–18.
49. Hunt T, Ferrar M, Miller L, et al. The effect of effort on baseline neuropsychological test scores in high school football athletes. Arch Clin Neuropsychol 2007;22: 615–21.
50. Echemendia R. Measurement issues in sports neuropsychology. National Academy of Neuropsychology Bulletin 2010;25(2):5–9.
51. Meehan W, Bachur R. Sport-related concussion. Pediatrics 2009;123:114–23.
52. Halstead M, Walter K. The Council on Sports Medicine and Fitness. Clinical report–sport related concussion in children and adolescents. Pediatrics 2010; 126:597–615.
53. Lovell M, Fazio V. Concussion management in the child and adolescent athlete. Curr Sports Med Rep 2008;7(1):12–5.
54. Grady M. Concussion in the adolescent athlete. Curr Probl Pediatr Adolesc Health Care 2010;40:154–69.
55. Salinas C, Webbe F, Devore T. The epidemiology of soccer heading in competitive youth players. J Clin Sports Psychol 2009;3:15–33.

56. McKeever C, Schatz P. Current issues in the identification, assessment, and management of concussions in sports-related injuries. Appl Neuropsychol 2003;10:4.
57. Kirkwood M, Yeates K, Wilson P. Pediatric sport-related concussion: a review of the clinical management of an oft-neglected population. Pediatrics 2006;117: 1359–71.
58. Barlow K, Crawford S, Stevenson A, et al. Epidemiology of post-concussion syndrome in pediatric mild traumatic brain injury. Pediatrics 2010;126:e374–81.
59. Moser R, Fryer A, Bernardinelli S. Youth sport concussion: a heads up on the growing public health concern. In: Webbe F, editor. The handbook of sports neuropsychology. New York (NY): Springer; 2010. p. 187–207.
60. Lincoln A, Caswell S, Almquist J, et al. Trends in concussion incidence in high school sports. Am J Sports Med 2011;39(5):958–63.

Subacute Concussion-Related Symptoms in Youth

Heidi K. Blume, MD, MPH*, Sylvia Lucas, MD, PhD,
Kathleen R. Bell, MD

KEYWORDS

• Concussion • Child • Subacute symptoms
• Postconcussive symptoms • Post-traumatic headache
• Post-concussive syndrome

Most athletes who experience a single sports-related concussion recover from the acute effects within a few weeks. However, a minority of children and adolescents with concussion experience symptoms for many weeks, or even months, after the injury.[1,2] Concern also exists that children may take longer to recover from concussion than adults,[3] and that symptoms, recovery patterns, and optimal treatment strategies may be different for children than adults. Subacute and chronic symptoms related to concussion are particularly concerning in children, because cognitive deficits, headache or neck pain, sleep dysfunction, and emotional dysregulation can affect school performance and social function at a critical period of development and maturation.

Postconcussive symptoms are divided into three major domains:

1. Somatic symptoms: including headache, nausea, photophobia, phonophobia, vision changes, sleep disturbance, and balance deficits.
2. Emotional disturbance: including irritability, apathy, depression, and anxiety.
3. Cognitive symptoms: including slow processing speed, attention deficits, impaired concentration, and poor performance on neuropsychological testing.

Some have previously questioned the existence of postconcussion syndrome in children,[4] but recent prospective controlled studies show that mild traumatic brain injury (mTBI) or concussion in children is associated with a constellation of postconcussive symptoms.[1,2,5] This article reviews the epidemiology of subacute symptoms after pediatric concussion and the current recommendations for the assessment and management of these symptoms in children and adolescents. However, any review of these subjects is limited by the fact that few long-term prospective controlled studies of outcome after concussion in adolescents, very few long-term

Division of Pediatric Neurology, Seattle Children's Hospital, B-5552 Sand Point Way Northeast, Seattle, WA 98105, USA
* Corresponding author.
E-mail address: heidi.blume@seattlechildrens.org

Phys Med Rehabil Clin N Am 22 (2011) 665–681
doi:10.1016/j.pmr.2011.08.007
1047-9651/11/$ – see front matter © 2011 Elsevier Inc. All rights reserved.

pmr.theclinics.com

studies of younger children with concussion, and no large controlled studies of management of subacute or chronic symptoms after concussion in children or adolescents have been performed.

EPIDEMIOLOGY OF POSTCONCUSSION SYMPTOMS IN YOUTH

Although few prospective, controlled studies have been performed specifically related to pediatric concussion in sports, several recent studies have examined postconcussive symptoms after mTBI treated in the emergency department and compared these with postconcussive symptoms after other injuries in children. In this field, the prevalence of postconcussion symptoms in an injured but nonconcussed population is important, because headache, irritability, sleep problems, and other subacute postconcussive symptoms are also common in the general population. Yeates and colleagues[2] found that, when parents were asked about these symptoms 1, 3, and 12 months after injury, children with mTBI were more likely to have a higher number of acute and persistent postconcussive symptoms than those who had experienced an orthopedic injury. In the acute period, within 3 weeks of injury, headache was the most commonly reported symptom (76%).

A controlled prospective study of mTBI in children (ages 1 month to 18 years) seen in the emergency department found that 11% of those with mTBI still had some complaints of postconcussive symptoms 3 months after their injury compared with 0.5% of those with extracranial injury (ECI). In children older than 6 years, 13.7% of those with mTBI and 1% of those with ECI were still symptomatic 3 months after injury. The most common postconcussive symptoms that were increased from baseline at 1 month after injury were fatigue (79%), "more emotional" (60%), irritability (58%), and headache (58%).[1] The comprehensive age range (1 month to 18 years) included in this study must be considered when evaluating these results in relation to sports-related concussion, because headache or other specific symptoms may be difficult for very young children to express to their parents, the pathophysiology of and recovery from mTBI are likely different in different age groups, and the mechanism of head injury may affect symptoms and recovery. The possibility that post-concussive symptoms may be related to age and injury severity is demonstrated by Barlow's finding that symptomatic children with mTBI were older than asymptomatic children and children with more severe mTBI had a significantly higher probability of remaining symptomatic over time. In this study 2.3% of those with mTBI remained symptomatic for longer than 12 months and 60% of these symptomatic children had chronic post-traumatic headache.[1]

Another controlled study comparing outcomes 3 months after mTBI and ECI (as part of a study examining an educational intervention for mTBI) found that mean postconcussive symptom scores were not different between the groups. However, 20% of the mTBI group had significant "ongoing difficulties" at 3 months after injury. These children tended to have a history of prior head injury, learning difficulties, other neurologic or psychiatric disturbance, or family stressors.[6]

In their study of postconcussive symptoms after pediatric mTBI (ages 8–15 years) or orthopedic injury treated in the emergency department, Taylor and colleagues investigated the time course of parental and child reports of somatic, cognitive, and emotional postconcussive symptoms after injury.[7] They found that higher parental counts of total postconcussive symptoms were associated with younger age at injury and female sex. Higher child ratings of somatic postconcussive symptoms were associated with lower socioeconomic status and female sex. They also found that somatic postconcussive symptom ratings were highest for mTBI acutely, then declined at 1 and 3 months and were not different from reports of those with orthopedic injury at 12 months. Ratings of cognitive postconcussive symptoms peaked at 3 months, and although these declined in both groups, they were still significantly different between mTBI and orthopedic injury groups at 12 months. Emotional postconcussive symptoms were associated only with preinjury postconcussive symptom ratings and were not significantly associated with mTBI.[7]

Studies of sports-related concussion provide further insight. Field and colleagues[3] found that high school athletes took significantly longer to recover to their expected performance level on neuropsychological testing after concussion (7 days) than college athletes (3 days). Athletes who reported 5 minutes or more of altered mental status with confusion or amnesia at the time of concussion were more likely to have longer-lasting memory deficits and complaints of postconcussive symptoms.[8,9] Concern also exists that prior concussion increases the risk of prolonged postconcussive symptoms after subsequent concussions. Even at baseline, high school athletes with a history of two or more concussions had significantly higher ratings of subacute concussion symptoms at baseline than athletes with a history of zero or one prior concussion, although all athletes had been free of acute concussion for at least 4 months before testing.[10] Lau and colleagues[11] found that self-reported cognitive decline, migraine symptoms, and slow ImPACT reaction time after concussion were each associated with prolonged recovery in high school athletes.

In summary, most children and adolescents recover to their preinjury baseline relatively quickly after concussion, but a few children experience prolonged symptoms. School-aged children and adolescents seem to be at higher risk for prolonged subacute symptoms after concussion than either very young children or college-aged adults. Other risk factors for prolonged postconcussive symptoms include more severe concussion and multiple past concussions. Learning disability, preexisting anxiety or depression, and presence of migraine or headaches before injury are also believed to be risk factors for prolonged symptoms after concussion,[11] although preexisting deficits can be difficult to differentiate from concussion-induced symptoms, and these factors have not been well studied after concussion in children or adolescents.

GENDER AND POSTCONCUSSIVE SYMPTOMS

The role of gender in risk of concussion and postconcussive symptoms is complex. Several studies have found that female athletes are at higher risk for concussion than male athletes participating in similar sports,[12,13] but data are conflicting regarding the role of sex in recovery from concussion in youth sports. Female sex was associated with a higher count of postconcussive symptoms in the months after pediatric mTBI (ages 8–15 years) evaluated in the emergency department.[7] Broshek and colleagues[14] found that female college and high school athletes were more likely to display cognitive deficits after concussion than males. However, other studies found no difference in return to play or duration of complaints of postconcussive symptoms between males and females but did find sex-related differences in the kinds of symptoms reported, and that female athletes performed significantly worse than male athletes on visual memory tasks after concussion.[15,16] Women and men also report different changes in postconcussive symptoms after exercise in general.[17] Preiss-Farzanegan and colleagues[18] describe a higher risk for several postconcussive symptoms 3 months after sports-related mTBI for adult women compared with men (including headache, dizziness, fatigue, irritability, concentration problems) but not for girls (ages 7–17 years) compared with boys. Complex interactions among age, sex, concussion, and postconcussive symptoms are likely, given that many biologic sex-related differences that may be associated with concussion risk and postconcussive symptom risk, including size, weight, muscle mass, strength, migraine risk, and hormonal milieu, become significant in adolescence.

GENERAL EVALUATION OF POSTCONCUSSIVE SYMPTOMS

As stated by many authors in this issue, athletes with a suspected concussion must be evaluated by a trained medical professional before considering returning to play. This evaluation should include directed questions regarding postconcussive symptoms. Many programs use some form of the Postconcussion Symptom Scale (PCSS). The athlete is asked to rate 22 symptoms, including somatic, emotional, and cognitive symptoms, on a 0- to 6-point scale (**Table 1**). Providers should ask the athlete and parent if physical or cognitive activity increases any of these symptoms. Athletes may not recognize signs of a concussion and may underreport symptoms,[19] and therefore these questions are important to address directly during the evaluation of an athlete after head trauma. The history should also include a detailed description of when and how the concussion occurred, presence and length of time of altered mental

Table 1
Postconcussion symptom scale

Current Symptoms	None	Mild		Moderate		Severe	
Headache	0	1	2	3	4	5	6
Pressure in head	0	1	2	3	4	5	6
Neck pain	0	1	2	3	4	5	6
Nausea/vomiting	0	1	2	3	4	5	6
Dizziness	0	1	2	3	4	5	6
Balance problems	0	1	2	3	4	5	6
Blurred vision	0	1	2	3	4	5	6
Sensitivity to light	0	1	2	3	4	5	6
Sensitivity to noise	0	1	2	3	4	5	6
Sleep pattern changes	0	1	2	3	4	5	6
Drowsiness	0	1	2	3	4	5	6
Feeling slowed down	0	1	2	3	4	5	6
Feeling "in a fog"	0	1	2	3	4	5	6
"Don't feel right"/not like yourself	0	1	2	3	4	5	6
Difficulty concentrating	0	1	2	3	4	5	6
Difficulty remembering/ forgetfulness	0	1	2	3	4	5	6
Fatigue or low energy	0	1	2	3	4	5	6
Confusion	0	1	2	3	4	5	6
Nervous or anxious	0	1	2	3	4	5	6
More emotional/ emotions feel "closer to the surface"	0	1	2	3	4	5	6
Irritability/frustration	0	1	2	3	4	5	6
Sadness	0	1	2	3	4	5	6

How do you feel currently? Please circle a number for each of the symptoms listed above.

status or amnesia following the concussion, number and timing of past concussions, time to recovery from past concussions, and questioning about presence of symptoms on the PCSS before injury. The provider also should note any history of learning disability, attention deficits, headache, or mental health issues in the athlete before the concussion, because these factors may influence the risk of prolonged recovery after concussion. The results of neuroimaging and other testing should be reviewed, particularly if neuropsychological or cognitive testing had been performed before the concussion. Use of a standardized evaluation format that includes the PCSS is helpful so that change in symptoms can be followed objectively at each visit to document recovery or conversion to chronic postconcussion syndrome.

PHYSICAL EXAMINATION FOR POSTCONCUSSIVE SYMPTOMS

The physical examination of a child with subacute postconcussive symptoms may be focused on the athlete's complaints but should include a comprehensive neurologic examination, including evaluation of cranial nerve function, orientation, concentration, memory, coordination, vision, and balance (using the Balance Error Scoring System[20]) and a physical examination of the head and neck to detect evidence of pain or muscular tension in the neck, shoulders, and head. Postconcussive symptoms may be from direct head trauma but may also be related to a whiplash-type injury, which may cause additional cervical pain and symptoms. Fundoscopic examination should also be performed to look for papilledema or other signs of increased intracranial pressure or significant intracranial injury.

What Not to Miss

In the acute stage after sports-related concussions, rare but life-threatening entities to consider include intracranial hemorrhage, epidural hematoma, cerebral edema, cervical spine injury, other acute intracranial injury and skull fracture. At the subacute stage, other rare but potentially dangerous syndromes to consider in the appropriate setting include vascular dissection with transient ischemic attack or stroke-like symptoms, intracranial venous thrombosis, subacute subdural hematoma, and cervical spine injury. Indications for neuroimaging include seizures, repeated emesis, prolonged period of altered mental status, loss of consciousness longer than 30 seconds, or focal abnormalities on neurologic examination.[21] The role of neuroimaging in concussion is addressed in greater detail by McCullough and Jarvik elsewhere in this issue. Use of drugs and alcohol should also be addressed, because 40% to 50% of high school students use alcohol regularly[22] and use of alcohol or other drugs may complicate assessment of and recovery from concussion.

MANAGEMENT OF SUBACUTE SYMPTOMS AFTER CONCUSSION
Rest

Current guidelines stress the need for physical and cognitive rest after concussion, with a gradual return to activity when patients are symptom-free[21,23] (see article on Return to Play by Laker and Herring elsewhere in this issue). Many athletes report that their postconcussive symptoms worsen with either cognitive or physical activity. To prevent exacerbation of symptoms, they may need to temporarily stay out of school, reduce the length of time in school, reduce their academic workload, be allowed more time to complete assignments, have note takers provided, and have testing expectations altered (see article by Gioia elsewhere in this issue). Cognitive rest should also include eliminating or limiting time spent using computers, video games, and television, because these activities require attention and concentration and may exacerbate postconcussive symptoms. Because of slower reaction times, teens may also need to temporarily avoid driving.[21]

After concussion, athletes should rest physically and not return to play until they are symptom-free at rest. Once athletes are symptom-free at rest, they should be directed to gradually return to activity, as outlined in the Consensus Statement on Concussion in Sport[23] and reviewed by Guskiewicz and by Laker and Herring elsewhere in this issue. However, evidence shows that low-impact subthreshold exercise that does not exacerbate symptoms is safe and may be beneficial for adolescents with slow recovery after concussion.[24,25]

Concussion Education

Education about what to expect after concussion and strategies to deal with postconcussive symptoms seems to have a beneficial effect on outcome. Ponsford and colleagues[6] studied an educational intervention for 130 children with mTBI; 61 received a booklet outlining symptoms associated with mTBI, the likely time course of postconcussive symptoms, and coping mechanisms to deal with these symptoms, and 58 mTBI controls received traditional treatment. At 3 months after injury, parents in the mTBI control group reported that their injured children had significantly more postconcussive symptoms than those in the educational intervention group. Specifically, the education group had fewer complaints of headaches, sleeping difficulties, and problems with judgment than the control group. The control group also tended to report greater irritability, inattentiveness, and conduct problems than the intervention group. However, the proportion of children with "significant ongoing problems" requiring referral for additional assistance was similar in the intervention and control groups (21% vs 19%).

SUBACUTE SYMPTOMS OF CONCUSSION

Although the guidelines for concussion management apply to concussion and postconcussive symptoms in general, many athletes have one or two symptoms that are particularly problematic and disabling. This article discusses the evaluation and management of several of the most common subacute postconcussive symptoms, including headache, sleep disturbance, balance deficits, and emotional changes. Cognitive changes after concussion are of vital importance and are addressed in greater detail by Goia, Cantu, and Coppel elsewhere in this issue.

Headache After Concussion

Headache is one of the most common symptoms after concussion, reported by 72% to 93%[1,26,27] of children and teens with concussion or mTBI. Blinman and colleagues[26] found that 32% of children reported headache 2 to 3 weeks after mTBI. A study of concussions reported in the High School Reporting Information Online database, found that although more than 90% of high school athletes who experienced concussion reported headache initially, 83% had resolution of all symptoms within 1 week and only 1.5% reported symptoms lasting longer than 1 month.[27] However, in a prospective controlled study of mTBI in children aged 1 month to 18 years of age, Barlow and colleagues[1] found that 58% reported headache 1 month after injury and 9 of 670 children (1.3%) had chronic headache 12 months after injury.

Posttraumatic headache (PTH) is defined by the *International Classification of Headache Disorders: 2nd Edition* as a secondary headache that develops within 7 days of head trauma (or regaining consciousness after traumatic brain injury).[28] Criteria are based on severity of injury, latency from injury, and duration of the headache. No descriptions of headache localization, characterization, or accompanying features are used. Several studies in adult civilian and military populations have attempted to classify headache using primary headache criteria.[29] Although few studies have addressed the classification of pediatric PTH, adult studies of PTH have found that migraine and probable migraine accounted for approximately 57% of the population with headache at 3 months, whereas tension-type and cervicogenic headache accounted for 18% and 6%, respectively. Approximately 31% were unclassifiable using these criteria.[30] Given that PTH and the primary headache disorders share many similar characteristics, some investigators have postulated that the migraine and PTH may have common pathophysiologic mechanisms, but the mechanisms of both syndromes remains unclear.[31,32]

Women seem to be at higher risk of headache after mTBI than men, but this association was not found for younger girls (ages 6–17 years).[15,18] In another study, female sex was associated with higher number of total and somatic postconcussive symptoms 3 months after mTBI, but the authors did not mention headache specifically.[33] A study of high school athletes found that headache was reported acutely after sports-related concussion in similar numbers of boys and girls (95% and 97%, respectively),[15] and found a difference in the types of postconcussive symptoms reported by boys and girls, but no difference was seen in the number of postconcussive symptoms reported between boys and girls.

Although sex-related differences in risk of headache after concussion have not been studied in detail in children or adolescents, primary headache disorders such as migraine are more common in women than men, and the difference in migraine prevalence between men and women becomes pronounced around the time of puberty.[34] Thus, if similarities exist between migraine and PTH, adolescent girls may be at higher risk for significant headache after concussion than boys. One study of PTH in an adult population, women were more likely to report headache 1 year after injury (37% vs 18%; $P<.01$).[30]

Preexisting migraine is thought to be a risk factor for significant PTH in adults, and in a study of PTH in adults after complicated mild to moderate or severe traumatic brain injury, individuals with preexisting headaches were more likely to report headache at 3, 6, and 12 months after traumatic brain injury compared with those without preexisting headache (45% vs 19%; $P<.001$).[30] This relationship has not been explored after pediatric concussion. In addition, we believe that family history of migraine may be a risk factor for significant headache after concussion, because concussion may trigger or unmask an underlying headache syndrome or predisposition to migraine in vulnerable populations, but this relationship has not been well studied.

Postconcussive headaches are associated with significant disability for student athletes, and several authors have found lower performance on neurocognitive testing for concussed athletes with migrainous headache compared with those without headaches or with nonmigrainous headaches.[9,35] However, whether the headaches are a sign of a more severe concussion or are directly causing disability is difficult to determine. Migraine headaches after concussion are also associated with balance abnormalities[36] and prolonged recovery time.[11] However, even migraine headaches not related to concussion can affect testing performance, attention, and memory[37,38] and therefore severe headache after concussion, particularly when combined with the other sequelae of concussion, may lead to pronounced difficulties with concentration, attention, cognition, and school performance.

One of the most difficult questions facing providers is whether the occurrence of headache should limit the athlete's activities, particularly if the athlete experienced some headache before concussion. Current guidelines suggest that athletes with persistent headache or headache exacerbated by physical activity should not return to play,[23] and the American Academy of Pediatrics suggests that athletes with symptoms lasting 3 months or longer after concussion should consider prolonged time away from sports.[21] Although the optimal management of headache after concussion not affected by activity is less clear, these athletes are likely to be at substantial risk for developing more significant and prolonged symptoms if they experience another concussion.

Management of headache after concussion
Physical and cognitive rest is the mainstay of initial concussion management,[23] and education about postconcussive symptoms may help improve outcome,[6] but no other randomized controlled studies of the treatment of concussion-related headaches in youth have been performed. Certainly, typical strategies for headache management should be used, emphasizing maintenance of good hydration, regular sleep, regular meals, and avoidance of triggers and excessive stress. However, few firm guidelines exist for pharmaceutical treatment of these headaches in pediatric or adult populations, except that nonsteroidal anti-inflammatory drugs should not be used if hemorrhage is a concern, and therefore treatment practice varies widely.

Most athletes will not require aggressive management of headaches after concussion. However, when an athlete develops prolonged or disabling headaches related to concussion, active headache management with medications may be considered. Athletes who experience PTH must follow the typical lifestyle guidelines listed earlier for headache management. Evidence suggests that if symptoms do not improve within 4 to 6 weeks after concussion, providers may consider recommending low-impact subthreshold exercise, defined as a progressive low-impact aerobic exercise program that does not exacerbate postconcussive symptoms[24,25] (such as walking, slow swimming, or stationary biking, and **not** to be confused with active "return to play" exercise). This strategy seems to be safe and may be beneficial for adolescents with prolonged symptoms after concussion.[24,25]

Many providers use the primary headache characteristics of the PTH to guide treatment, and may try medications typically used for primary headache disorders to manage disabling or prolonged posttraumatic headaches. Once intracranial hemorrhage has been excluded through imaging or clinical parameters, use of ibuprofen, naproxen, and acetaminophen to control headaches in the first few weeks after concussion has been discussed.[39] Sumatriptan, a 5-HT1B/1D agonist postulated to block release of calcitonin gene-related peptide and other inflammatory neuropeptides, preventing neurogenic inflammation and causing vasoconstriction of dural-based meningeal arteries, has been used to successfully treat acute PTH.[40] However, patients and providers must set limits on use of over-the-counter analgesics, caffeine-containing compounds, opiates, and triptans to avoid the potential complication of medication overuse.

Physical therapy or massage therapy may also be helpful in the management of PTH, particularly in the presence of cervical muscular tenderness or strain. Biofeedback and behavioral therapies are often helpful in the management of adult and pediatric headache,[41,42] but this has not been studied in pediatric PTH. If patients have a chronic disabling headache with cervical or occipital tenderness, trigger point injections or nerve blocks administered by experienced providers in appropriate circumstances may be considered.

Many different medications have been used to help manage frequent PTH. Amitriptyline a tricyclic antidepressant, is one of the most commonly recommended by medical providers.[39] It is frequently used to treat primary headache disorders in children and adolescents and may help manage comorbid insomnia and sleep disruption in patients with concussion, although it may exacerbate excessive sleepiness and cognitive dysfunction. A few small studies in adults found that amitriptyline may be effective treatment for PTHs, but studies in children are lacking.[43] Topiramate is another commonly used medication for pediatric headache, and providers discuss its use in postconcussive headaches. However, concerns exist that topiramate may worsen concussion-related cognitive deficits in susceptible patients.

A small informal survey of pediatric headache specialists found that many medications are considered for the management of prolonged problematic headache after concussion, including amitriptyline, topiramate, magnesium, valproic acid, steroids, dihydroergotamine, gabapentin, propranolol, and selective serotonin reuptake inhibitors, although amitriptyline was the most commonly mentioned medication (American Headache Society: Pediatric & Adolescent Headache Section, personal communication of members of this group to H. Blume, 2011). This list of medications is similar to that outlined in a recent review of medical treatment of concussion.[39] In some refractory cases, a combination of therapies may be most effective. However, the choice of medication and therapy will depend on the patient's symptoms, history, and comorbidities. The use of daily medication to manage headache after concussion should only be considered by experienced and trained practitioners when an athlete has a disabling headache that is not following the expected course of improvement after concussion.

Sleep Disorders After Concussion

Complaints about sleep quality and quantity are frequent after concussion, as are complaints about fatigue, which may not be associated with poor sleep. A lack of restorative sleep may contribute to worsening of other postconcussion symptoms or disorders, such as headache, trouble concentrating, and depression.

A short review of sleep mechanisms can illustrate why sleep may be affected after concussion. Both sleep, defined as a natural and periodic state of rest during which consciousness of the world is suspended, and wake, defined as a state of alertness, are important concepts that have distinct neurophysiologic underpinnings. Normal sleep includes the states of sleep, defined by the presence or absence of rapid eye movements (rapid eye movement [REM] and non–rapid eye movement [NREM], respectively) and circadian rhythms. These aspects of normal sleep are different for children and adolescents compared with adults. In NREM sleep, muscles are not paralyzed and mental activity is fragmented, although dreaming is rare. Stage N3 of NREM sleep is characterized by deep slow wave sleep, and is when parasomnias such as sleep-walking most often occur. REM sleep is characterized by muscle atonia and dreaming, and comprises 20% to 25% of the sleep cycle.

The circadian rhythm is an approximately 24-hour cycle that, although regulated internally, is highly responsive to external stimuli such as light and is independent of prior sleep/wake duration. In addition, sleep has a homeostatic aspect, in that the longer one is awake, the sleepier one becomes. Conversely, the longer one sleeps, the less "pressure" they have to remain asleep. Areas of the brain that are key for initiating and maintaining sleep include the suprachiasmatic nucleus in the hypothalamus (affecting pineal gland secretion of melatonin) and the brainstem areas (eg, laterodorsal tegmental and pediculopontine tegmental nuclei, dorsal raphe nuclei, nucleus locus ceruleus). Wakefulness also is affected by the dorsal raphe and locus ceruleus and by neurons located in the lateral hypothalamus, projecting to the brainstem and forebrain areas that secrete hypocretin, a peptide that promotes wakefulness and inhibits REM sleep.

Sleep is essential to normal cognition, and disordered sleep can result in further impairment of cognition after concussion. During wakefulness, the brain can actively interact with the external world, accumulating information and experience. In NREM sleep, the brain is actively "off-line," and investigators believe that repetitive activity recorded as spindle and K complexes on electroencephalogram may be a reiteration of inputs that enhance memory consolidation. During REM sleep, the brain is reactivated with different patterns of regional blood flow and microchemistry that integrate recently stored memories with other stored memories during the dreaming process. Areas particularly activated with dreaming include the ventromedial and dorsolateral prefrontal cortex, the anterior limbic structures, and the inferior parietal and visual association areas in the posterior cortex.

Sleep characteristics change normally as children grow. Adolescents have the greatest rate and number of changes. Overall need for sleep decreases by a few hours, but the need for REM sleep remains the same. As puberty progresses, a change in circadian rhythms occurs with later onset of sleep. Latency of sleep often decreases and there is more perception of sleepiness. Sleep disorders in children may be associated with disordered nighttime breathing, external social influences, depression, academic challenges, impaired attention, and mood disturbances.[44]

Approximately 30% to 60% of persons complain of disordered sleep after traumatic brain injury, including insomnia, hypersomnia, respiratory associated disorders, and circadian rhythm disorders. Insomnia is defined as difficulty initiating or maintaining sleep for at least 1 month accompanied by subjective impairment in daytime functioning. Ouellet and colleagues[45] reported that 50% of persons with traumatic brain injury reported insomnia symptoms and almost 30% met criteria for insomnia syndrome. Among the cases of insomnia, 60% were severe and chronic. Factors associated with this included mTBI, fatigue, depression, and pain. Fichtenberg and colleagues[46] reported insomnia in similar proportions of hospitalized patients with traumatic brain injury. Sleep disorders seem to be more common among patients with moderate to severe traumatic brain injury than among uninjured controls, with 80% complaining of insomnia symptoms compared with 23%, respectively.[47] These symptoms seem to be long-lasting; those with persistent insomnia complaints also had greater neurobehavioral impairments and worse occupational outcomes.[48] Although fatigue is a common complaint among those with traumatic brain injury, it is likely to be multifactorial, with insomnia, pain, depression, and cognitive effort all contributing to the perception of fatigue.

Sleep apnea may also be more common after traumatic brain injury. For patients in an inpatient rehabilitation unit, disordered respiration was more common (36%) than would be predicted by age norms.[49,50] Studies using polysomnography have produced mixed results, with some finding discrepancies between self-reports of sleep disturbance and polysomnographic findings. Circadian rhythm disturbances are often misinterpreted as insomnia. Ayalon and colleagues reported that 15 of 24 patients with traumatic brain injury and complaints of insomnia actually had circadian rhythm sleep disorder.[51] Complaints of daytime sleepiness may be associated with low hypocretin levels.[52,53]

Few studies describe sleep in children and adolescents after sports-related concussions or other types of mTBI. After mTBI, children ages 12 to 17 reported that excess sleep was the most common postconcussive symptom in the postacute period (36%), whereas difficulties falling asleep were the most severe symptom.[27] However, for children and adolescents with mTBI, polysomnographic findings are mixed. In one study, reports of sleep difficulties did not correlate with polysomnographic findings.[54] Another study described lower sleep efficiency, more awakenings, and more wake time in adolescents with mTBI.[55]

Management of sleep disorders after concussion

Management of sleep disorder can be particularly challenging in adolescents with concussion. The disorder must be defined first to ensure that associated factors, such as pain, depression, or respiratory disorders, are addressed. Inquiring about pre-injury and family sleep patterns is also useful. A sleep diary may be helpful to outline prebedtime activities, use of caffeine or alcohol, and the sleep environment. No specific interventions have been well studied for sleep disorders after concussion. However, it is reasonable to first address sleep hygiene, including banning television or computer use before bedtime, restricting caffeine use, and encouraging aerobic exercise during the daytime and a dark, quiet sleep environment. Ouellet and Morin[56] successfully used cognitive–behavioral treatment in a small group of persons with traumatic brain injury to improve sleep efficiency and reduce symptoms of fatigue. Graduated bedtime/wake time adjustments, the use of melatonin, and bright light therapy may be useful in circadian rhythm sleep disorders. Caution is highly recommended regarding the use of sedative-hypnotics in children and adolescents to treat insomnia (**Table 2**).

Balance Disturbances After Concussion

Balance disturbances are common immediately after concussion at all ages. Disordered balance after concussion has several potential causes, including central and peripheral mechanisms. However, most data exist for college-age athletes, and very few studies address younger children. None of the current balance screens used for postconcussion testing have been normed for children younger than 16 years, and children do not reach adult levels for visual and vestibular afferent function until approximately age 15 to 16 years.[57,58]

Table 2
Comparative normal sleep characteristics for children and adolescents

	Sleep Stages	Required Number of Hours	Awakenings	Sleep Difficulties
Children (ages 5–12 y)	—	Age 5 y: 11 Age 12 y: 9.5	2	20%–41% (parasomnias: chronic in 1%–6%; bedtime resistance)
Adolescents and teens	Decreased stage 3/4 non–rapid eye movement sleep	9–10	—	Increased sleepiness, excessive somnolence, increased sleep latency, awakenings, movement during sleep, delayed sleep phase disorder (7%)

Data from Millman RP. Excessive sleepiness in adolescents and young adults: causes, consequences, and treatment strategies. Pediatrics 2005;115(6):1774–86; and Carno MA, Hoffman LA, Carcillo JA, et al. Developmental stages of sleep from birth to adolescence, common childhood sleep disorders: overview and nursing implications. J Pediatr Nurs 2003;18(4):274–83.

College-age football players return to normal levels of balance within 5 to 10 days.[59,60] Persons with mTBI have increased reliance on visual inputs for balance and are less able to use vestibular orienting information on balance testing.[61] As with many other features of concussion, college-age players with slower symptom resolution also show more persistent signs of postural instability.[62] In addition, as noted earlier, college athletes with persisting posttraumatic headache had worse scores for balance and other physical tests after concussion.[36]

Few studies of younger children after concussion or mTBI exist. Gagnon and colleagues[63] noted that children with mTBI (with a mean Glasgow Coma Score of 14.8) without persisting balance complaints showed abnormalities on postural testing compared with controls. These findings were particularly notable during testing when vision was occluded and for postural tasks requiring higher levels of coordination. In fact, other authors have noted that postural stability testing may be more sensitive if the athlete is concurrently performing a cognitive task.[64]

Children with persisting balance disorders after concussion seem to respond to vestibular rehabilitation treatment, as do adults.[65]

Cognitive Symptoms After Concussion

The risk of subacute and long-term cognitive deficits associated with sports-related concussion is one of the most concerning topics for athletes, parents, providers and researchers. Cognitive symptoms such as slowed processing speed, memory impairment, poor attention, and confusion are common after concussion. Detailed neuropsychological testing often shows mild deficits even after athletes feel they are back to baseline, providing evidence for the value of including baseline and post-injury neurocognitive assessment in the complete assessment of the concussed athlete. In addition, athletes with a history of two or more prior concussions have lower scores on baseline testing than those without concussion,[10] although whether those with lower scores are more prone to concussion or if multiple concussions lead to poorer scores on testing is unclear. Given the significance of questions regarding subacute and long-term cognitive assessment and cognitive change after concussion, these complex questions are addressed in greater detail in three different articles by Goia, Cantu, and Coppel elsewhere in this issue.

Treatment of cognitive deficits after concussion may involve modification of school expectations for several weeks or even months, and support from teachers, school counselors, and family (see the article by Goia elsewhere in this issue). Fortunately, most athletes do not experience significant long-term cognitive deficits after a single concussion. However, the individuals who do experience long-lasting symptoms may benefit from consideration of further therapy. Small trials examining the use of stimulants, such as methylphenidate, after pediatric traumatic brain injury have shown equivocal results.[39] The use of amantadine to improve cognitive function has also been studied after more significant traumatic brain injury. However, the risks of these medications generally far outweigh the possible benefits for most children and adolescents with sports-related concussion.

Mood After Concussion

Athletes may develop emotional dysregulation after concussion and experience irritability, sadness, and emotional lability. Athletes who experience prolonged symptoms after concussion are at risk for mood or behavioral changes for many reasons including: a direct result of their concussion, difficulty coping with other symptoms, restriction from participation in their sport (either temporarily or permanently), modification of future plans that centered on athletics, and the loss of identity as an athlete.

Complaints of mood changes after concussion are common. Barlow and colleagues[1] report that at 1 month after injury, 60% of children with mTBI were more emotional and 58% were more irritable than baseline. In the acute period after pediatric mTBI, Blinman and colleagues[26] described complaints of sadness in 34% of children, nervousness in 44%, irritability in 40%, and feeling more emotional in 41%. A few weeks after mTBI, fewer children had emotional symptoms, including sadness in 19%, nervousness in 22%, irritability in 30%, and feeling more emotional in 25%.

In studies of adults with mTBI, those with depression or anxiety and mTBI have more postconcussive symptoms and tend to have longer duration of symptoms than those without these comorbid factors.[66,67] However, Taylor and colleagues[7] did not find a significant correlation between mTBI and emotional postconcussive symptoms, but did find a correlation between emotional postconcussive symptoms and preinjury emotional distress. Depression and anxiety in the absence of traumatic brain injury are also often associated with symptoms reported on the postconcussion checklist, including cognitive complaints, somatic complaints, and sleep disturbance. Thus, although depression or other mood changes after concussion should be addressed, some of these complaints may be related to preinjury factors in addition to factors associated with the concussion.

For most athletes, significant emotional dysregulation after concussion is short-lived and should be addressed with discussion of coping strategies, understanding and support from family and friends, and counseling with a trained therapist if needed.[39] However, occasionally these athletes may benefit from medical management of their symptoms with an experienced medical provider, particularly if other factors are contributing to their emotional symptoms, such as prolonged absence or retirement from sports or other preexisting emotional problems or family issues. Although no trials of medication or other therapy for depression related to concussion in children or adolescents have been performed, tricyclic antidepressants and serotonin reuptake inhibitors have been recommended for treating depression related to traumatic brain injury in adults.[39] However, medical management of emotional problems after concussion should only be considered by an experienced provider when the symptoms are not following the expected course of improvement.

SUMMARY

Fortunately, most youth do not experience prolonged somatic, cognitive, or emotional symptoms after sports-related concussion. However, current evidence indicates that younger athletes may have a longer recovery period than collegiate athletes, and that females may have a higher risk for more significant postconcussive symptoms than males. Given that millions of athletes experience concussions annually in the United States, if even a small fraction of concussed youth have prolonged or disabling subacute postconcussive symptoms, then thousands of young athletes and their families must deal with symptoms that interfere with critical academic, cognitive, and social development each year. Further rigorous research is essential to determine which athletes are at greatest risk for disability after concussion and to develop treatment strategies to minimize disability and promote a full recovery in children and adolescents after concussion.

ACKNOWLEDGMENTS

This paper was supported in part by the Department of Education, National Institute on Disability and Rehabilitation Research, TBI Model Systems: University of Washington Traumatic Brain Injury Model System H133A070032.

REFERENCES

1. Barlow KM, Crawford S, Stevenson A, et al. Epidemiology of postconcussion syndrome in pediatric mild traumatic brain injury. Pediatrics 2010;126(2): e374–81.
2. Yeates KO, Taylor HG, Rusin J, et al. Longitudinal trajectories of postconcussive symptoms in children with mild traumatic brain injuries and their relationship to acute clinical status. Pediatrics 2009;123(3):735–43.
3. Field M, Collins MW, Lovell MR, et al. Does age play a role in recovery from sports-related concussion? A comparison of high school and collegiate athletes. J Pediatr 2003;142(5):546–53.
4. Nacajauskaite O, Endziniene M, Jureniene K, et al. The validity of post-concussion syndrome in children: a controlled historical cohort study. Brain Dev 2006;28(8):507–14.
5. Ponsford J, Willmott C, Rothwell A, et al. Cognitive and behavioral outcome following mild traumatic head injury in children. J Head Trauma Rehabil 1999; 14(4):360–72.
6. Ponsford J, Willmott C, Rothwell A, et al. Impact of early intervention on outcome after mild traumatic brain injury in children. Pediatrics 2001;108(6): 1297–303.
7. Taylor HG, Dietrich A, Nuss K, et al. Post-concussive symptoms in children with mild traumatic brain injury. Neuropsychology 2010;24(2):148–59.
8. Lovell MR, Collins MW, Iverson GL, et al. Recovery from mild concussion in high school athletes. J Neurosurg 2003;98(2):296–301.
9. Collins MW, Field M, Lovell MR, et al. Relationship between postconcussion headache and neuropsychological test performance in high school athletes. Am J Sports Med 2003;31(2):168–73.
10. Schatz P, Moser RS, Covassin T, et al. Early indicators of enduring symptoms in high school athletes with multiple previous concussions. Neurosurgery 2011; 68(6):1562–7.
11. Lau B, Lovell MR, Collins MW, et al. Neurocognitive and symptom predictors of recovery in high school athletes. Clin J Sport Med 2009;19(3):216–21.
12. Covassin T, Swanik CB, Sachs ML. Sex differences and the incidence of concussions among collegiate athletes. J Athl Train 2003;38(3):238–44.
13. Gessel LM, Fields SK, Collins CL, et al. Concussions among United States high school and collegiate athletes. J Athl Train 2007;42(4):495–503.
14. Broshek DK, Kaushik T, Freeman JR, et al. Sex differences in outcome following sports-related concussion. J Neurosurg 2005;102(5):856–63.
15. Frommer LJ, Gurka KK, Cross KM, et al. Sex differences in concussion symptoms of high school athletes. J Athl Train 2011;46(1):76–84.
16. Covassin T, Schatz P, Swanik CB. Sex differences in neuropsychological function and post-concussion symptoms of concussed collegiate athletes. Neurosurgery 2007;61(2):345–50 [discussion: 50–1].
17. Gaetz MB, Iverson GL. Sex differences in self-reported symptoms after aerobic exercise in non-injured athletes: implications for concussion management programmes. Br J Sports Med 2009;43(7):508–13.
18. Preiss-Farzanegan SJ, Chapman B, Wong TM, et al. The relationship between gender and postconcussion symptoms after sport-related mild traumatic brain injury. PM R 2009;1(3):245–53.
19. Delaney JS, Lacroix VJ, Leclerc S, et al. Concussions among university football and soccer players. Clin J Sport Med 2002;12(6):331–8.

20. Riemann BL, Guskiewicz KM, Shields EW. Relationship between clinical and forceplate measures of postural stability. J Sport Rehabil 1999;8:71–82.
21. Halstead ME, Walter KD. American Academy of Pediatrics. Clinical report—sport-related concussion in children and adolescents. Pediatrics 2010;126(3):597–615.
22. Miller JW, Naimi TS, Brewer RD, et al. Binge drinking and associated health risk behaviors among high school students. Pediatrics 2007;119(1):76–85.
23. McCrory P, Meeuwisse W, Johnston K, et al. Consensus Statement on Concussion in Sport: the 3rd International Conference on Concussion in Sport held in Zurich, November 2008. Br J Sports Med 2009;43(Suppl 1):i76–90.
24. Gagnon I, Galli C, Friedman D, et al. Active rehabilitation for children who are slow to recover following sport-related concussion. Brain Inj 2009;23(12):956–64.
25. Leddy JJ, Kozlowski K, Donnelly JP, et al. A preliminary study of subsymptom threshold exercise training for refractory post-concussion syndrome. Clin J Sport Med 2010;20(1):21–7.
26. Blinman TA, Houseknecht E, Snyder C, et al. Postconcussive symptoms in hospitalized pediatric patients after mild traumatic brain injury. J Pediatr Surg 2009;44(6):1223–8.
27. Meehan WP III, d'Hemecourt P, Comstock RD. High school concussions in the 2008-2009 academic year: mechanism, symptoms, and management. Am J Sports Med 2010;38(12):2405–9.
28. Headache Classification Subcommittee of the International Headache Society. The international classification of headache disorders: 2nd edition. Cephalalgia 2004;24(Suppl 1):9–160.
29. Theeler BJ, Flynn FG, Erickson JC. Headaches after concussion in US soldiers returning from Iraq or Afghanistan. Headache 2010;50(8):1262–72.
30. Hoffman JM, Lucas S, Dikmen S, et al. Natural history of headache following traumatic brain injury. J Neurotrauma 2011;28:1719–25.
31. Lenaerts ME, Couch JR, Couch JR. Posttraumatic headache. Curr Treat Options Neurol 2004;6(6):507–17.
32. Packard RC. Chronic post-traumatic headache: associations with mild traumatic brain injury, concussion, and post-concussive disorder. Curr Pain Headache Rep 2008;12(1):67–73.
33. Bazarian JJ, Blyth B, Mookerjee S, et al. Sex differences in outcome after mild traumatic brain injury. J Neurotrauma 2010;27(3):527–39.
34. Stewart WF, Lipton RB, Celentano DD, et al. Prevalence of migraine headache in the United States. Relation to age, income, race, and other sociodemographic factors. JAMA 1992;267(1):64–9.
35. Mihalik JP, Stump JE, Collins MW, et al. Posttraumatic migraine characteristics in athletes following sports-related concussion. J Neurosurg 2005;102(5):850–5.
36. Register-Mihalik JK, Mihalik JP, Guskiewicz KM. Balance deficits after sports-related concussion in individuals reporting posttraumatic headache. Neurosurgery 2008;63(1):76–80 [discussion: 2].
37. O'Bryant SE, Marcus DA, Rains JC, et al. The neuropsychology of recurrent headache. Headache 2006;46(9):1364–76.
38. Meyer JS, Thornby J, Crawford K, et al. Reversible cognitive decline accompanies migraine and cluster headaches. Headache 2000;40(8):638–46.
39. Meehan WP III. Medical therapies for concussion. Clin Sports Med 2011;30(1):115–24, ix.
40. Abend NS, Nance ML, Bonnemann C. Subcutaneous sumatriptan in an adolescent with acute posttraumatic headache. J Child Neurol 2008;23(4):438–40.

41. Baumann RJ. Behavioral treatment of migraine in children and adolescents. Paediatr Drugs 2002;4(9):555–61.
42. Hermann C, Blanchard EB. Biofeedback in the treatment of headache and other childhood pain. Appl Psychophysiol Biofeedback 2002;27(2):143–62.
43. Tyler GS, McNeely HE, Dick ML. Treatment of post-traumatic headache with amitriptyline. Headache 1980;20(4):213–6.
44. Millman RP. Excessive sleepiness in adolescents and young adults: causes, consequences, and treatment strategies. Pediatrics 2005;115(6):1774–86.
45. Ouellet MC, Beaulieu-Bonneau S, Morin CM. Insomnia in patients with traumatic brain injury: frequency, characteristics, and risk factors. J Head Trauma Rehabil 2006;21(3):199–212.
46. Fichtenberg NL, Zafonte RD, Putnam S, et al. Insomnia in a post-acute brain injury sample. Brain Inj 2002;16(3):197–206.
47. Parcell DL, Ponsford JL, Rajaratnam SM, et al. Self-reported changes to nighttime sleep after traumatic brain injury. Arch Phys Med Rehabil 2006;87(2):278–85.
48. Cohen M, Oksenberg A, Snir D, et al. Temporally related changes of sleep complaints in traumatic brain injured patients. J Neurol Neurosurg Psychiatry 1992;55(4):313–5.
49. Webster JB, Bell KR, Hussey JD, et al. Sleep apnea in adults with traumatic brain injury: a preliminary investigation. Arch Phys Med Rehabil 2001;82(3):316–21.
50. Castriotta RJ, Lai JM. Sleep disorders associated with traumatic brain injury. Arch Phys Med Rehabil 2001;82(10):1403–6.
51. Ayalon L, Borodkin K, Dishon L, et al. Circadian rhythm sleep disorders following mild traumatic brain injury. Neurology 2007;68(14):1136–40.
52. Baumann CR, Bassetti CL. Hypocretins (orexins) and sleep-wake disorders. Lancet Neurol 2005;4(10):673–82.
53. Baumann CR, Werth E, Stocker R, et al. Sleep-wake disturbances 6 months after traumatic brain injury: a prospective study. Brain 2007;130(Pt 7):1873–83.
54. Korinthenberg R, Schreck J, Weser J, et al. Post-traumatic syndrome after minor head injury cannot be predicted by neurological investigations. Brain Dev 2004; 26(2):113–7.
55. Kaufman Y, Tzischinsky O, Epstein R, et al. Long-term sleep disturbances in adolescents after minor head injury. Pediatr Neurol 2001;24(2):129–34.
56. Ouellet MC, Morin CM. Efficacy of cognitive-behavioral therapy for insomnia associated with traumatic brain injury: a single-case experimental design. Arch Phys Med Rehabil 2007;88(12):1581–92.
57. Steindl R, Kunz K, Schrott-Fischer A, et al. Effect of age and sex on maturation of sensory systems and balance control. Dev Med Child Neurol 2006;48(6):477–82.
58. Schneiders AG, Sullivan SJ, Gray AR, et al. Normative values for three clinical measures of motor performance used in the neurological assessment of sports concussion. J Sci Med Sport 2010;13(2):196–201.
59. McCrea M, Guskiewicz KM, Marshall SW, et al. Acute effects and recovery time following concussion in collegiate football players: the NCAA Concussion Study. JAMA 2003;290(19):2556–63.
60. Peterson CL, Ferrara MS, Mrazik M, et al. Evaluation of neuropsychological domain scores and postural stability following cerebral concussion in sports. Clin J Sport Med 2003;13(4):230–7.
61. Rubin AM, Woolley SM, Dailey VM, et al. Postural stability following mild head or whiplash injuries. Am J Otol 1995;16(2):216–21.
62. Slobounov S, Slobounov E, Sebastianelli W, et al. Differential rate of recovery in athletes after first and second concussion episodes. Neurosurgery 2007;61(2): 338–44 [discussion: 44].

63. Gagnon I, Swaine B, Friedman D, et al. Children show decreased dynamic balance after mild traumatic brain injury. Arch Phys Med Rehabil 2004;85(3): 444–52.
64. Parker TM, Osternig LR, VAN Donkelaar P, et al. Gait stability following concussion. Med Sci Sports Exerc 2006;38(6):1032–40.
65. Alsalaheen BA, Mucha A, Morris LO, et al. Vestibular rehabilitation for dizziness and balance disorders after concussion. J Neurol Phys Ther 2010;34(2):87–93.
66. Lange RT, Iverson GL, Rose A. Depression strongly influences postconcussion symptom reporting following mild traumatic brain injury. J Head Trauma Rehabil 2011;26(2):127–37.
67. McCauley SR, Boake C, Levin HS, et al. Postconcussional disorder following mild to moderate traumatic brain injury: anxiety, depression, and social support as risk factors and comorbidities. J Clin Exp Neuropsychol 2001;23(6):792–808.

Long-Term Consequences: Effects on Normal Development Profile After Concussion

Daniel H. Daneshvar, MA[a],*, David O. Riley, SB[a],
Christopher J. Nowinski, AB[a,b], Ann C. McKee, MD[c],
Robert A. Stern, PhD[a], Robert C. Cantu, MD[a,b,d,e,f]

KEYWORDS

- Concussion • Development
- Chronic traumatic encephalopathy
- Postconcussion syndrome • Youth

In the United States, approximately 1.7 million people sustain a traumatic brain injury (TBI) annually; these injuries account for 1.365 million emergency room visits and 275,000 hospitalizations each year.[1] The majority of these TBIs are minor, with 75% of these injuries classified as mild TBIs (mTBI) or concussions.[2] These numbers

This work was supported by the Boston University Alzheimer's Disease Center NIA P30 AG13846, supplement 0572063345-5, the National Operating Committee on Standards for Athletic Equipment, the National Collegiate Athletic Association, the National Federation of State High School Associations, the American Football Coaches Association, and the Sports Legacy Institute.

The authors have nothing to disclose.

[a] Department of Neurology, Center for the Study of Traumatic Encephalopathy (CSTE), Boston University School of Medicine (BUSM), 72 East Concord Street, B7800, Boston 02118, MA, USA
[b] Sports Legacy Institute, PO Box 181225, Waltham, MA, USA
[c] Department of Neurology, Center for the Study of Traumatic Encephalopathy (CSTE), Bedford VA Hospital, Boston University School of Medicine (BUSM), 200 Springs Road, 182-B, Boston, MA 01730, USA
[d] Department of Neurosurgery, Neurologic Sports Injury Center, Brigham and Women's Hospital, 5 Francis Street, Boston, MA, USA
[e] Department of Surgery, Emerson Hospital,131 Old Road to Nine Acre Corner, Concord, MA, USA
[f] Department of Neurosurgery, Center for the Study of Traumatic Encephalopathy (CSTE), Boston University School of Medicine (BUSM), John Cuming Building, Suite 820, 131 ORNAC, Concord, MA 01742, USA
* Corresponding author.
E-mail address: ddanesh@bu.edu

may, however, vastly underestimate the total incidence of concussion, as many individuals suffering from mild or moderate TBI do not seek medical advice, especially in the 81% to 92% of cases when the concussion is not accompanied by loss of consciousness.[1,3–5] Beyond the burden of the injury itself, these TBIs have significant direct and indirect economic consequences, estimated at more than $60 billion annually in the United States alone.[6]

A concussion is a brain injury caused by a force transmitted to the head from a direct or indirect contact with the head, face, neck, or elsewhere, which results either in a collision between the brain and skull or in a strain on the neural tissue and vasculature.[7,8] This impact or strain is believed to cause the symptoms of concussion through a cascade characterized by abrupt neuronal depolarization, release of excitatory neurotransmitters, ionic shifts, altered glucose metabolism and cerebral blood flow, and impaired axonal function.[8] Although these injuries are known to cause short-term deficits, the long-term effects of this neuropathologic cascade are less defined.[9–14]

Clinically the acute signs and symptoms of a concussion are similar in children and adults, and can include physical signs (eg, loss of consciousness, amnesia), behavioral changes (eg, irritability), cognitive impairment (eg, slowed reaction times), sleep disturbances (eg, drowsiness), somatic symptoms (eg, headaches), cognitive symptoms (eg, feeling "in a fog"), and/or emotional symptoms (eg, emotional lability).[15] These deficits are observed in the absence of structural brain damage in diagnostic magnetic resonance imaging (MRI).[16,17] While the vast majority of these symptoms resolve spontaneously, many others may linger.[9] In addition, no two concussions have the same presentation or identical outcomes.[18]

The specific mechanism underlying neural tissue damage, however, appears to be different in the adult versus the developing brain.[19,20] While severe TBI has been shown to have both serious and long-term consequences on personality, mood, and cognition, the precise effect of concussions on development has yet to be fully elucidated.[21–27] Furthermore, immature neural tissue differs from mature tissue in response to injury, in terms of both plasticity and altered developmental trajectory.[28] The structure of the brain, in relation to the skull and its musculature, is also dissimilar in adults and children, leading to different biomechanics and thus different injury profiles.[29,30] As a result, different presentations and outcomes would be expected in response to a concussion experienced in youth as compared with one experienced as an adult.

LONG-TERM EFFECTS OF POSTCONCUSSION SYNDROME

The symptoms of a concussion may take some time to resolve, resulting in significant long-term burden. When the symptoms of concussion persist as a variety of cognitive, somatic, and behavioral changes, these lingering deficits comprise postconcussion syndrome (PCS).[17,31–33] PCS is defined by the *International Classification of Diseases, 10th Revision* (ICD-10) as the occurrence within 1 month of injury of at least 3 of the 8 symptom categories listed in **Box 1**.[34] The *Diagnostic and Statistical Manual of Mental Disorders* (Fourth Edition, Text Revised) (DSM-IV-R) requires the presence of symptoms in at least 3 of 6 categories for at least 3 months after injury in addition to evidence of neuropsychological dysfunction, as outlined in **Box 2**.[35] Whether PCS is experienced following an mTBI seems to be dependent on a combination of factors, including premorbid vulnerability, postinjury psychological adjustment, and postinjury changes in brain function.[36] While most of these symptoms typically resolve within a few days or weeks following mTBI or other head injury, some individuals suffer from PCS for months or longer and, although studies remain conflicting, it is believed

---

Box 1
Characteristics of postconcussion syndrome according to the ICD-10

History of head trauma with loss of consciousness precedes symptom onset by maximum of 4 weeks

Three or more symptom categories:

- Headache, dizziness, malaise, fatigue, noise intolerance

- Irritability, depression, anxiety, emotional lability

- Subjective concentration, memory, or intellectual difficulties without neuropsychological evidence of marked impairment

- Insomnia

- Reduced alcohol intolerance

Preoccupation with above symptoms and fear of brain damage with hypochondriacal concern and adoption of sick role

Data From World Health Organization. The ICD-10 classification of mental and behavioral disorders: diagnostic criteria for research. Geneva (Switzerland): World Health Organization; 1993.

---

that as many as 15% of people with a history of mTBI still suffer from deficits 1 year after injury.[17,37,38]

Adults with PCS often initially present with physical symptoms such as dizziness and headache in the first weeks following injury, with psychosocial symptoms such as depression and irritability first appearing up to a month later.[39] These findings mimic those of rodent models, which have reported both impaired learning and

---

Box 2
Characteristics of postconcussion syndrome according to the DSM-IV-R

A history of head trauma that has caused significant cerebral concussion (eg, with loss of consciousness, posttraumatic amnesia, or seizures)

Neuropsychological evidence of difficulty in attention or memory

Three or more symptoms that last at least 3 months and have an onset shortly after head trauma or represent substantial worsening of previous symptoms:

- Fatigue

- Disordered sleep

- Headache

- Dizziness

- Irritability or aggression with little or no provocation

- Anxiety, depression, or affect lability

- Changes in personality

- Apathy or lack of spontaneity

The symptoms result in significant impairment in daily functioning that reflects a decline from previous level

Data from American Psychiatric Association. Diagnostic and statistical manual of mental disorders. 4th edition. Washington, DC: American Psychiatric Association; 1994.

---

depressive-like behavior in mice following mTBI, perhaps mediated by apoptotic cell death.[40–42] In addition, single and repeated concussions in adults have been shown to be correlated with cognitive deficits months following the injury.[43] Executive functioning impairment also appears to persist, with adults who had experienced an mTBI 6 months prior found to have significantly decreased information processing speed.[44] At 1 year after injury, the most common symptoms appear to be a combination of the physical, the psychosocial, and the cognitive, with reports of headaches, dizziness, disturbances of senses, light and noise sensitivity, and various psychiatric symptoms, including depression, anxiety, coping issues, and psychosocial disability.[45,46] In addition, studies have suggested that women are more likely to develop PCS, in terms of both more symptoms reported and a longer duration of impairment.[47]

Some adults continue to show motor deficits, functional deficits, and persistent depressive symptoms more than 1 year after injury.[48–50] The data here are conflicting, however, with other studies indicating that neuropsychological deficits appear to resolve by 1 year after injury. These latter studies tend to include all individuals who had been exposed to any mTBI rather than just those who experienced PCS symptoms; as a result, the sample is overly dilute and the resulting lack of association is not surprising.[51–54]

Of interest, several studies have looked at how beliefs regarding expected outcome in response to brain injury might influence an individual's risk of developing PCS. One study found that individuals who had suffered an mTBI and who indicated that they believed their symptoms would have serious negative consequences on their lives were significantly more likely to experience PCS at 3 months following the injury. In fact, these beliefs regarding the perceived severity at the time of injury were more predictive of PCS symptoms at 3 months than were the total number of PCS symptoms reported immediately following the injury.[45] Another study evaluating attitudes surrounding injury recovery found that self-ratings of PCS symptoms were positively related to emotion-focused coping strategies and negatively related to problem-focused coping in adults who had experienced an mTBI.[55] These findings suggest that one's attitudes can influence the extent to which a concussion has long-term, persistent effects.

Although PCS is considered to be fully recoverable with proper treatment, suffering from PCS-related symptoms for an extended time may delay an individual's return to work, adversely affect one's quality of life, and result in additional social and economic costs.[17,31,45] The deficits caused by these symptoms may also have an indirect long-term effect by exacerbating a preexisting depression or impairing the ability to adequately cope with stress.[56–58] In addition, there is some evidence that concussions result in chronic motor and neuropsychological changes over 3 decades following injury[59]; however, these findings may be attributable to an early-stage neurodegenerative disease associated with concussion, as discussed later.

Although studies and diagnostic criteria of PCS initially reported dissimilar symptoms for adult and pediatric populations, it is now acknowledged that children and young adults report a PCS that is similar to adults and may suffer from the same behavioral, emotional, and somatic difficulties following mTBI.[36,60] Many of these initial studies of youth concussions focused on athletes, as they tend to be at increased risk of experiencing concussions.[5] Although college football athletes report a higher incidence of concussion than high school athletes, it has been reported that high school athletes take longer to recover, based on neuropsychological testing.[61] This finding of increased youth susceptibility to PCS has been extended to other sports and activities, and is perhaps explained by the fact that the frontal lobes do not fully develop until late adolescence.[43] Rodent models have also suggested that the immature brain is more susceptible than the adult brain to apoptosis following mTBI.[62,63] In fact, one prospective cohort study found that age at the time of injury and extent of extracranial injury were the two strongest independent predictors of functional outcome at 6 months after injury.[64] Even in young adults well enough to enroll and continue in college, there is evidence that PCS symptoms may last for years, and that there may be gender differences in PCS resolution, with women reporting more lingering mood and anxiety symptoms.[65]

Children differ significantly from adults and adolescents not only in size but also biomechanically, pathophysiologically, neurobehaviorally, and developmentally.[28] Because the developing brain is more plastic than the mature brain, younger age at the time of injury was originally thought to have a beneficial effect on recovery and expected outcome.[66] However, current literature indicates that this is not the case; the developing brain appears, in fact, to be more vulnerable to diffuse brain injury. Traumatic injury to the immature brain results in a prolonged period of pathogenesis in both cortical and subcortical structures, leading to progressive neurodegeneration, hyperactivity, and sustained cognitive impairments.[67,68]

Although early studies showed either a small or no effect of head injuries on the developing brain, many of these studies had flawed designs; less than half of the 56 studies reviewed by Satz and colleagues[69,70] from 1970 through 1998 met even 4 of the 6 following recommendations for methodologically sound studies: (1) the inclusion of control groups (either with no injury or with other body injury); (2) the use of a longitudinal design with follow-up assessment post injury; (3) a clear definition of mild injury, without the inclusion of children with more severe injuries; (4) the inclusion of at least 20 children with mTBI; (5) the use of standardized tests to measure outcomes; and (6) controls for preinjury risk factors.

The most methodologically sound studies have found that children report worse cognitive symptoms more than 1 year after concussion than adults. These deficits are first reported months after the original injury and affect the child's school work or abilities to function at home.[71] Children aged 6 to 12 years with mTBI have impaired executive functioning and attention 1 year after injury compared with noninjured controls.[72] An mTBI may also cause linguistic changes that adversely affect Verbal IQ and expressive language. Of note, although these deficiencies improved by 6 months after injury, no additional improvement was observed between 6 and 24 months.[73] In such cases where symptoms persist, PCS may adversely affect a child's conduct and personality, and can lead to extended school absence and limitations on athletic play. In fact, one study reported that children who showed more PCS symptoms displayed worse overall adjustment in comparison with children with fewer PCS symptoms.[36] It has also been suggested that individuals with higher cognitive ability have better outcomes following head injury, because they may be able to recruit alternative and additional neural substrates to compensate for tissue damage.[71,74,75]

Although animal models have elucidated the general pathophysiology responsible for acute concussive symptoms, the underlying cause of sustained PCS remains a matter of debate. However, several pathologic mechanisms have been proposed. Some make the pathophysiologic case that a contributing factor for sustained PCS is the microstructural damage of the brain from head injury. Given that the acute injury causes the aforementioned pathophysiologic cascade, it is not unlikely that some of the resulting microstructural damage can persist in some cases and result in the persisting symptoms of PCS sometimes observed.[31] However, as already mentioned for mTBI in adults, the correlation between increased risk of sustained PCS in children with negative coping strategies or beliefs about their mTBI symptoms indicates that there may also be a psychopathologic cause to this long-term PCS.[45,55]

This matter is further complicated by various methodologic shortcomings in mTBI and PCS research.[76] These limitations may include retrospective, cross-sectional designs, a lack of appropriate control groups, and a failure to separate different degrees of PCS.[36,39] In addition, studies rely heavily on the self-report of postconcussive symptoms by patients; this has a history of being unreliable, and studies show that a patient's self-report may be the result of simple malingering, an involvement in litigation, or recall biases such as the "good old days" bias, the idea that individuals who sustain an injury often underestimate problems preinjury.[17,77] Finally, whereas PCS is an acknowledged condition, there is a disagreement between ICD-10 and DSM-IV diagnostic criteria; this disagreement emphasizes the confusion over the underlying cause of long-term PCS. Whereas the ICD-10 criteria classifies PCS as symptoms without neuropsychological impairment and focuses instead on premorbid conditions and postinjury psychological adjustment, the DSM-IV criteria do require this neuropsychological impairment and seem to assume that PCS and related symptoms are at least partially caused by an underlying brain trauma.[78] The variability in diagnostic criteria, and the assumptions about PCS that this variation implies, result in different incidence estimates and limited diagnostic agreement when dealing with PCS patients.[79]

The enduring effects of PCS appear to be a combination of the biologic, the physiologic, the psychological, and the social. For both the pediatric and adult population, future research that incorporates genetics, advanced neuroimaging, refined cognitive and postconcussive symptom measures, and social environment research can help to achieve an integrated "biopsychosocial" model that may aid in the management of long-term PCS.[78] This, along with effective education and rehabilitation of patients, will work to reduce the incidence and burden of long-term PCS in TBI patients.

EFFECTS ON BEHAVIOR

Having sustained a previous concussion may alter a child's long-term developmental trajectory years after the symptoms of PCS subside. Studies of PCS typically only follow children for up to 1 year after injury, potentially before the full effects of the injury have manifested themselves. As a result, these studies are unable to measure the extent of the long-term detrimental effects of an mTBI on the developing brain. To properly evaluate the long-term consequences of youth concussion, studies must examine cognitively mature individuals who previously experienced a concussion in their youth.[80]

Because the prefrontal cortex is one of the last brain structures to mature, it is not surprising that parents report attention deficits, hyperactivity, or conduct disorder following a head injury to their child.[60] In addition, it has been shown that the number of long-term neurobehavioral symptoms in children is related to the severity of the initial mTBI as well as the child's neuropsychological functioning, academic performance, emotional adjustment, and adaptive functioning.[36,81]

The majority of previous studies examining the effects of brain injuries on development years after the injury have focused on more severe injuries.[82–85] However, these studies of moderate and severe TBI suggest a specific window of time during which the brain may be more vulnerable to injury; TBI experienced in middle childhood and later appears to be less detrimental than injuries sustained earlier.[86–91]

One cohort study of 490 children who experienced an mTBI before age 14 years, and who had no prior history of psychiatric illness, found that these children were significantly more likely to have psychiatric issues in the 3 years following injury than were uninjured controls. The children most commonly presented with attentional problems in the first year following injury. However, there was no difference observed in children who had already had a prior history of psychiatric illness in the year preceding the injury.[92]

These studies are complicated by the fact that the children more likely to experience concussions were also more likely to have undiagnosed psychiatric issues. To circumvent this issue, some studies have used detailed retrospective questionnaires to assess preinjury psychiatric status. One prospective longitudinal study found that children who experienced an mTBI requiring hospitalization before age 10 years displayed increased hyperactivity/inattention and conduct disorder between the ages of 10 and 13 compared with children who had not experienced an mTBI, as rated both by their mothers and their teachers.[89] This cohort has been followed through age 16, and these issues have been shown to persist.[93] However, these children did not display any deficits in intelligence or academic skills. In addition, children whose injuries did not require hospitalization showed no differences from control children without a history of mTBI. Although there were differences observed in hyperactivity/inattention and conduct disorder based on age at the time of injury (those injured between 0 and 5 years old and those injured between 5 and 10 years old), these differences were not statistically significant.[89] A later study confirmed these findings and also reported that children injured in preschool had progressively worsening parent and teacher ratings of hyperactivity/inattention and conduct disorder when followed longitudinally from age 7 to 13 years.[80] Another study of 45 adults, with an average age at injury of 8.9 years (standard deviation of 3.3), found that those who experienced posttraumatic amnesia for at least 30 minutes had statistically significant decreases in measures of attention and memory more than 2 decades later.[94] These attentional findings are not surprising, as the prefrontal cortex does not fully develop until late adolescence. In addition, these deficits were not observed in individuals injured as adults.[95]

The effects of mTBI on children do not always end with the resolution of PCS, but may have long-term effects on cognitive processing, mood, and behavior. These delayed behavioral impairments suggest the need for continued monitoring and intervention in children, even years after initial concussion.

WHEN TO RETIRE AFTER A CONCUSSION

Following a concussion, the absolute contraindications to return to a contact/collision practice or competition sport include:

1. Abnormal neurologic assessment
2. Symptomatic of postconcussion signs/symptoms at rest or exertion
3. If done, neuropsychological battery not baseline or above
4. If done, head computed tomography or MRI shows a lesion placing the athlete at increased risk of head injury (edema, hemorrhage, hydrocephalus, cavum septum pellucidum, arachnoid cyst).

The relative contraindications to return to collision practice or competition include:

1. Postconcussion symptoms that last many months and not days
2. Mild or indirect blows (whiplash) that produce significant and lengthy postconcussion symptoms.

Thus there are absolute and relative indicators for retirement. Neither are based on a particular number of concussions, but rather on the athlete's response, including duration of symptoms and ease of being concussed. Keeping in mind the increased vulnerability of the developing brain, it is suggested that one might be even more conservative in the under-18 age group as compared with adults.[96]

DEGENERATIVE DISEASE

Brain trauma has long been thought to play a role in initiating or accelerating the molecular cascade involved in several degenerative diseases, including Alzheimer disease (AD), Parkinson disease (PD), and amyotrophic lateral sclerosis (ALS).[97–99] In addition, repetitive concussive and subconcussive brain trauma has been implicated as the primary risk factor for developing the progressive neurodegenerative disease chronic traumatic encephalopathy (CTE), as well as the motor neuron disease variant chronic traumatic encephalomyelopathy (CTE-M).[100,101]

Alzheimer Disease

Several epidemiologic studies have found a relationship between head trauma and AD in later life.[102–108] However, all of these studies based their analyses on a clinical diagnosis of possible or probable AD. Without neuropathologic confirmation of disease, it is possible that other neurodegenerative diseases, such as CTE, were in fact partially or fully responsible for the observed clinical dementia.[109] However, one retrospective study found that individuals with a history of TBI had a higher than expected prevalence of AD pathology observed at autopsy.[110] This result could in part be explained by the fact that β-amyloid precursor protein (APP) is shown to temporarily accumulate in response to acute TBI in genetically susceptible mice; the cleavage of APP results in the β-amyloid (Aβ) characteristic of AD.[111,112] More research is certainly needed, both to elucidate the relationship between AD and mTBI, and to disambiguate potential cases of CTE from clinically diagnosed cases of probable and possible AD.

Parkinson Disease

TBI has also been implicated as a risk factor for PD.[98,113] Although the nature of the relationship is poorly understood, animal models suggest that TBI results in α-synuclein deposition, a protein shown to be the primary building block of the Lewy bodies in PD.[112,114,115] However, neither animal models nor human studies have conclusively shown a relationship between concussions and the development of PD.

Chronic Traumatic Encephalopathy

CTE is a progressive neurodegenerative tauopathy caused by repeated concussive and subconcussive impacts. Because repeated impacts are thought to be necessary to initiate the disease process, CTE is typically found in those at high risk for experiencing repetitive head trauma, including athletes, those with exposure to injury due to military service or occupation, and individuals who exhibit seizures and/or head-banging behavior.[100,109] In fact, CTE was initially named dementia pugilistica because of its association with the repetitive head trauma experienced by boxers in the ring.

However, head trauma alone is not sufficient to initiate the neuropathologic cascade of CTE. There are many potential risk factors that likely play a role in determining which individuals develop CTE and which individuals do not, given similar head trauma histories. There is some evidence that the ApoE E4 allele may be associated with CTE development.[100,101] In addition, the relationship between the development of CTE and the number or severity of head injuries is not yet clear, as some athletes diagnosed with CTE had no reported concussion history despite a history of repetitive subconcussive head trauma.[100,101] In addition, the age at which an individual begins experiencing head injury and the time interval between concussions may play a role in the development of CTE.

Although the disease process likely starts at the time of injury, the initial signs of CTE do not typically manifest until decades later. Therefore, the time course for the presentation of CTE symptoms distinguish it from the cumulative effects of multiple injuries or a form of prolonged PCS. CTE can only be diagnosed post mortem at this time, and as such the precise clinical presentation and the cascade of events preceding it are not yet known.[116] In addition, because the diagnosis of CTE relies on postmortem tissue analysis, the precise epidemiology of CTE is not yet known. Although the majority of professional and collegiate athletes examined for CTE have in fact been found to have had the disease, this represents a biased sample in that families who suspect their loved ones may be impaired are more likely to agree to brain donation for research purposes.

However, CTE is believed to be characterized clinically by a progressive decline of memory and executive functioning; mood and behavioral disturbances that include depression, apathy, impulsivity, anger, irritability, suicidal behavior, and aggressiveness; gait changes that resemble Parkinsonism; and, eventually, progression to dementia. Once this disease process is initiated, the neurodegeneration typically progresses slowly, with a mean survival duration of 18 years following the onset of symptoms.[100,117–119]

CTE is characterized neuropathologically by a distinctive pattern of extensive tau-immunoreactive inclusions scattered throughout the cerebral cortex in a patchy, superficial distribution, with focal epicenters at the depths of sulci and around the cerebral vasculature; extensive tau-immunoreactive inclusions in limbic and paralimbic regions as well as brainstem nuclei; and a relative absence of Aβ deposits. On gross examination, CTE is characterized by generalized atrophy and enlarged ventricles, specific atrophy of the frontal and medial temporal lobes, degenerations of white matter fiber bundles, cavum septum pellucidum often with fenestrations, thinning of the hypothalamic floor, and shrinkage of the mammillary bodies.[100]

Although CTE may have similarities with AD, they are two quite distinct diseases. Clinically, CTE typically presents with age of onset in the 40s and 50s as opposed to onset after age 65 years in sporadic AD. In addition, the clinical progression of disease is much slower, often lasting decades, and is characterized by a subtle deterioration in personality and behavior.[100] Neuropathologically both diseases share tau immunoreactivity, but the widespread distribution of neurofibrillary and glial tangles in the frontal, insular, and temporal cortices, white matter, diencephalon, brainstem, and spinal cord is considerably more extensive in CTE than in AD. Furthermore, the pattern of the neurofibrillary abnormalities is entirely distinct from AD or any other tauopathy, especially when considering the absence of the neuritic Aβ deposits characteristic of AD.[100,120] However, additional research is needed to better understand the mechanism underlying these changes.

Motor Neuron Disease

Although genetic mutations have been identified that cause ALS, 90% to 95% of ALS cases are sporadic.[121,122] Many risk factors have been identified as possibly contributing to these sporadic cases, but trauma specifically has been implicated as a risk factor that may initiate the molecular cascades resulting in ALS.[99,123] In one case-control study, researchers found that injuries that had occurred in the previous 10 years had the strongest association with diagnosis of ALS.[99] Another case-control study also found that the risk of ALS increased when the last head injury occurred closer to the time of diagnosis.[124] However, other studies have disputed this association.[125] On the whole, these findings suggest that head injury may play a role in triggering the onset of motor neuron disease.

Motor neurons in sporadic ALS are often found with TDP-43–immunoreactive inclusion bodies that appear either as rounded hyaline inclusions or as skein-like inclusions; as a result, TDP-43 has been implicated in the pathogenesis of motor neuron disease.[126,127] Widespread TDP-43–positive inclusions have also been found in the vast majority of cases of CTE, and are typically found in the brainstem, basal ganglia, diencephalon, medial temporal lobe, frontal, temporal, and insular cortices, and subcortical white matter. A subset of individuals with CTE also develops a progressive motor neuron disease characterized by profound weakness, atrophy, spasticity, and fasciculations. In these individuals, both tau neurofibrillary pathology and extensive TDP-43–immunoreactive inclusions and neurites were found in the motor cortex of the brain and in the spinal cord in a distribution not characteristic of sporadic ALS.[101] Although these initial findings merit further investigation, the co-occurrence of widespread TDP-43 and tau proteinopathies in CTE suggests that repetitive head injury might be associated with the deposition of two abnormally phosphorylated, misfolded proteins, and that in some individuals the TDP-43 proteinopathy is associated with the development of a motor neuron disease.

IMPLICATIONS ON ATHLETIC PARTICIPATION

As a result of these potential long-term consequences, both the incidence and the severity of youth concussion must be reduced. There are several approaches worth evaluating toward this end.

One potential solution involves the development and introduction of better equipment (eg, helmets and mouth guards) that are specifically designed to attenuate the forces associated with concussions. However, although helmets have been shown to decrease the incidence of facial injury as well as moderate and severe TBI, and mouth guards help protect against dental and orofacial injury, there has been no evidence to date that the newest equipment reduces the incidence of concussions or severity of concussion symptoms.[5]

In addition, when new equipment requirements are introduced into a sport, athletes' behavior often changes, resulting in a riskier style of play reflecting their increased feeling of protection.[128] In some cases, this has been associated with a paradoxic increase in concussion incidence within an activity.[129]

A potentially more fruitful approach would be to limit an athlete's exposure to the impacts that might result in concussion. This goal could be accomplished through several means, such as decreasing the number of contact practices an athlete participates in each week; practice alone is responsible for up to 1500 impacts of 10 g or more for some football players.[130] Ivy League colleges have taken the lead and recently began implementing this policy, and it is hoped that others will follow suit. In addition, sport-specific rule changes might help reduce the frequency of unnecessary and dangerous collisions, thereby decreasing the burden of athletic concussion.

In most instances, when concussions are properly treated they are not believed to be associated with any long-term sequelae. Ensuring that individuals receive proper medical care, and are given adequate physical and mental rest during recovery, should ensure that these injuries fully heal. Adopting uniform return-to-play guidelines, such as those already discussed here, would help ensure athletes are not permitted to play too soon.

Along these lines, proper education of athletes, coaches, medical professionals, and the general public is necessary to identify and properly treat concussions. There are many organizations, such as the Centers for Disease Control and Prevention, the Brain Injury Association, and the Sports Legacy Institute, working to improve concussion awareness and educational outreach.

SUMMARY

While most concussions fully resolve within weeks of the injury, for some these concussions can have serious, long-term effects. Concussed individuals can sometimes experience prolonged PCS, lasting for months or even years, which can result in significant physical, emotional, and cognitive stress. In addition, in children and young adults, months of PCS can adversely affect one's developmental trajectory by keeping students out of class and straining personal relationships. In adults, suffering from PCS for an extended period of time may delay one's ability to return to work, resulting in an additional financial and social burden on the concussed individual.

Once the symptoms of concussion subside, in some cases a prior concussion may also have a lasting effect on behavior. These issues are more common in children, as those who have been concussed are more likely to have symptoms of mood or conduct disorders reported by parents and teachers years after injury. Although these findings may in part be due to undiagnosed mood or conduct disorders in children, which resulted in an original injury, the fact that the prefrontal cortex has not fully developed in these injured children provides an additional explanation of aberrant behavior.

In addition, concussions and subconcussive impacts have been shown to increase the risk of developing degenerative disease, sometimes even decades after the injury. There is a good deal of epidemiologic evidence linking a history of head injury with the development of AD, supported by evidence from animal models in response to acute head injury, but additional work is necessary to separate clinically diagnosed AD from other dementias. TBI has also been linked to PD through transient increases in α-synuclein resulting in an increase in the formation of Lewy bodies. However, the strongest evidence for a direct link between repetitive concussive and subconcussive injury and neurodegenerative disease later in life comes from the study of CTE. Originally found in boxers, CTE has been diagnosed in a wide variety of individuals, all of whom had been exposed to repetitive head injury, be it through participation in athletics, military service, occupational hazards, or some other cause. While the tau diagnostic of CTE may begin to aggregate and form inclusions as early as in the second decade, the first clinical signs of CTE are not typically observed until one's 30s or 40s. CTE presents with cognitive deficits, depression, and behavioral disinhibition, and eventually progresses to full-blown dementia.

Although concussions were once considered relatively benign, mounting evidence indicates that concussions can have long-term consequences, sometimes for years or even decades after the injury. Improved understanding of the risks associated with concussions, and their potentially debilitating consequences, highlights the need for better diagnosis, treatment, and prevention.

REFERENCES

1. Faul M, Xu L, Wald MM, et al. Traumatic brain injury in the United States: emergency department visits, hospitalizations and deaths 2002–2006. Washington, DC: US Department of Health and Human Services; 2010.
2. CDC. Report to Congress on mild traumatic brain injury in the United States: steps to prevent a serious public health problem. Atlanta (GA): National Center for Injury Prevention and Control; 2003.

3. Langlois JA, Rutland-Brown W, Wald MM. The epidemiology and impact of traumatic brain injury: a brief overview. J Head Trauma Rehabil 2006;21(5):375–8.
4. CDC. Nonfatal traumatic brain injuries from sports and recreation activities—United States, 2001–2005. Atlanta (GA): Centers for Disease Control and Prevention; 2007.
5. Daneshvar DH, Nowinski CJ, McKee AC, et al. The epidemiology of sport-related concussion. Clin Sports Med 2011;30(1):1–17, vii.
6. Finkelstein E, Corso P, Miller T. The incidence and economic burden of injuries in the United States. New York: Oxford University Press; 2006.
7. Concussion (mild traumatic brain injury) and the team physician: a consensus statement. Med Sci Sports Exerc 2006;38(2):395–9.
8. Barkhoudarian G, Hovda DA, Giza CC. The molecular pathophysiology of concussive brain injury. Clin Sports Med 2011;30(1):33–48, vii–iii.
9. Cantu RC, Herring SA, Putukian M. Concussion. N Engl J Med 2007;356(17): 1787 [author reply: 1789].
10. Covassin T, Stearne D, Elbin R. Concussion history and postconcussion neurocognitive performance and symptoms in collegiate athletes. J Athl Train 2008;43(2):119–24.
11. Belanger HG, Vanderploeg RD. The neuropsychological impact of sports-related concussion: a meta-analysis. J Int Neuropsychol Soc 2005;11(4):345–57.
12. McCrea M, Guskiewicz KM, Marshall SW, et al. Acute effects and recovery time following concussion in collegiate football players: the NCAA Concussion Study. JAMA 2003;290(19):2556–63.
13. Bailes JE, Cantu RC. Head injury in athletes. Neurosurgery 2001;48(1):26–45 [discussion: 45–6].
14. Nolin P. Executive memory dysfunctions following mild traumatic brain injury. J Head Trauma Rehabil 2006;21(1):68–75.
15. McCrory P, Meeuwisse W, Johnston K, et al. Consensus statement on concussion in sport—the 3rd International Conference on concussion in sport, held in Zurich, November 2008. J Clin Neurosci 2009;16(6):755–63.
16. Davis GA, Iverson GL, Guskiewicz KM, et al. Contributions of neuroimaging, balance testing, electrophysiology and blood markers to the assessment of sport-related concussion. Br J Sports Med 2009;43(Suppl 1):i36–45.
17. Hall RC, Chapman MJ. Definition, diagnosis, and forensic implications of postconcussional syndrome. Psychosomatics 2005;46(3):195–202.
18. Cantu RC. Return to play guidelines after a head injury. Clin Sports Med 1998; 17(1):45–60.
19. Teasdale GM, Murray GD, Nicoll JA. The association between APOE epsilon4, age and outcome after head injury: a prospective cohort study. Brain 2005; 128(Pt 11):2556–61.
20. Shah SA, Prough DS, Garcia JM, et al. Molecular correlates of age-specific responses to traumatic brain injury in mice. Exp Gerontol 2006;41(11):1201–5.
21. Cantu RC, Guskiewicz K, Register-Mihalik JK. A retrospective clinical analysis of moderate to severe athletic concussions. PM R 2010;2(12):1088–93.
22. Levin HS, Song J, Ewing-Cobbs L, et al. Word fluency in relation to severity of closed head injury, associated frontal brain lesions, and age at injury in children. Neuropsychologia 2001;39(2):122–31.
23. Temkin NR, Corrigan JD, Dikmen SS, et al. Social functioning after traumatic brain injury. J Head Trauma Rehabil 2009;24(6):460–7.
24. Bombardier CH, Fann JR, Temkin NR, et al. Rates of major depressive disorder and clinical outcomes following traumatic brain injury. JAMA 2010;303(19): 1938–45.

25. Taylor HG, Swartwout MD, Yeates KO, et al. Traumatic brain injury in young children: postacute effects on cognitive and school readiness skills. J Int Neuropsychol Soc 2008;14(5):734–45.
26. Gerrard-Morris A, Taylor HG, Yeates KO, et al. Cognitive development after traumatic brain injury in young children. J Int Neuropsychol Soc 2010;16(1):157–68.
27. Anderson V, Catroppa C, Morse S, et al. Recovery of intellectual ability following traumatic brain injury in childhood: impact of injury severity and age at injury. Pediatr Neurosurg 2000;32(6):282–90.
28. Kirkwood MW, Yeates KO, Wilson PE. Pediatric sport-related concussion: a review of the clinical management of an oft-neglected population. Pediatrics 2006;117(4):1359–71.
29. Prins ML, Hovda DA. Developing experimental models to address traumatic brain injury in children. J Neurotrauma 2003;20(2):123–37.
30. Cantu RC, Mueller FO. The prevention of catastrophic head and spine injuries in high school and college sports. Br J Sports Med 2009;43(13):981–6.
31. Sterr A, Herron KA, Hayward C, et al. Are mild head injuries as mild as we think? Neurobehavioral concomitants of chronic post-concussion syndrome. BMC Neurol 2006;6:7.
32. Gosselin N, Tellier M. Patients with traumatic brain injury are at high risk of developing chronic sleep-wake disturbances. J Neurol Neurosurg Psychiatry 2010;81(12):1297.
33. Sojka P, Stalnacke BM, Bjornstig U, et al. One-year follow-up of patients with mild traumatic brain injury: occurrence of post-traumatic stress-related symptoms at follow-up and serum levels of cortisol, S-100B and neuron-specific enolase in acute phase. Brain Inj 2006;20(6):613–20.
34. WHO. The ICD-10 classification of mental and behavioural disorders: diagnostic criteria for research. Geneva (Switzerland): WHO; 1993.
35. APA. Diagnostic and statistical manual of mental disorders. 4th edition. Washington, DC: APA; 1994.
36. Yeates KO, Luria J, Bartkowski H, et al. Postconcussive symptoms in children with mild closed head injuries. J Head Trauma Rehabil 1999;14(4):337–50.
37. Carroll LJ, Cassidy JD, Peloso PM, et al. Prognosis for mild traumatic brain injury: results of the WHO Collaborating Centre Task Force on Mild Traumatic Brain Injury. J Rehabil Med 2004;(Suppl 43):84–105.
38. Rees PM. Contemporary issues in mild traumatic brain injury. Arch Phys Med Rehabil 2003;84(12):1885–94.
39. Yang CC, Tu YK, Hua MS, et al. The association between the postconcussion symptoms and clinical outcomes for patients with mild traumatic brain injury. J Trauma 2007;62(3):657–63.
40. Milman A, Rosenberg A, Weizman R, et al. Mild traumatic brain injury induces persistent cognitive deficits and behavioral disturbances in mice. J Neurotrauma 2005;22(9):1003–10.
41. Tashlykov V, Katz Y, Volkov A, et al. Minimal traumatic brain injury induces apoptotic cell death in mice. J Mol Neurosci 2009;37(1):16–24.
42. Tweedie D, Milman A, Holloway HW, et al. Apoptotic and behavioral sequelae of mild brain trauma in mice. J Neurosci Res 2007;85(4):805–15.
43. Wall SE, Williams WH, Cartwright-Hatton S, et al. Neuropsychological dysfunction following repeat concussions in jockeys. J Neurol Neurosurg Psychiatry 2006;77(4):518–20.
44. Johansson B, Berglund P, Ronnback L. Mental fatigue and impaired information processing after mild and moderate traumatic brain injury. Brain Inj 2009; 23(13–14):1027–40.

45. Whittaker R, Kemp S, House A. Illness perceptions and outcome in mild head injury: a longitudinal study. J Neurol Neurosurg Psychiatry 2007;78(6):644–6.
46. Panayiotou A, Jackson M, Crowe SF. A meta-analytic review of the emotional symptoms associated with mild traumatic brain injury. J Clin Exp Neuropsychol 2010;32(5):463–73.
47. Farace E, Alves WM. Do women fare worse: a metaanalysis of gender differences in traumatic brain injury outcome. J Neurosurg 2000;93(4):539–45.
48. Pagulayan KF, Hoffman JM, Temkin NR, et al. Functional limitations and depression after traumatic brain injury: examination of the temporal relationship. Arch Phys Med Rehabil 2008;89(10):1887–92.
49. Bell KR, Hoffman JM, Temkin NR, et al. The effect of telephone counselling on reducing post-traumatic symptoms after mild traumatic brain injury: a randomised trial. J Neurol Neurosurg Psychiatry 2008;79(11):1275–81.
50. Heitger MH, Jones RD, Dalrymple-Alford JC, et al. Motor deficits and recovery during the first year following mild closed head injury. Brain Inj 2006;20(8):807–24.
51. Dikmen SS, Corrigan JD, Levin HS, et al. Cognitive outcome following traumatic brain injury. J Head Trauma Rehabil 2009;24(6):430–8.
52. Straume-Naesheim TM, Andersen TE, Dvorak J, et al. Effects of heading exposure and previous concussions on neuropsychological performance among Norwegian elite footballers. Br J Sports Med 2005;39(Suppl 1):i70–7.
53. Broglio SP, Ferrara MS, Piland SG, et al. Concussion history is not a predictor of computerised neurocognitive performance. Br J Sports Med 2006;40(9):802–5 [discussion: 802–5].
54. Collie A, McCrory P, Makdissi M. Does history of concussion affect current cognitive status? Br J Sports Med 2006;40(6):550–1.
55. Woodrome SE, Yeates KO, Taylor HG, et al. Coping strategies as a predictor of post-concussive symptoms in children with mild traumatic brain injury versus mild orthopedic injury. J Int Neuropsychol Soc 2011;17(2):1–10.
56. Killam C, Cautin RL, Santucci AC. Assessing the enduring residual neuropsychological effects of head trauma in college athletes who participate in contact sports. Arch Clin Neuropsychol 2005;20(5):599–611.
57. Sawchyn JM, Brulot MM, Strauss E. Note on the use of the Postconcussion Syndrome Checklist. Arch Clin Neuropsychol 2000;15(1):1–8.
58. Machulda MM, Bergquist TF, Ito V, et al. Relationship between stress, coping, and postconcussion symptoms in a healthy adult population. Arch Clin Neuropsychol 1998;13(5):415–24.
59. De Beaumont L, Theoret H, Mongeon D, et al. Brain function decline in healthy retired athletes who sustained their last sports concussion in early adulthood. Brain 2009;132(Pt 3):695–708.
60. Mittenberg W, Wittner MS, Miller LJ. Postconcussion syndrome occurs in children. Neuropsychology 1997;11(3):447–52.
61. Field M, Collins MW, Lovell MR, et al. Does age play a role in recovery from sports-related concussion? A comparison of high school and collegiate athletes. J Pediatr 2003;142(5):546–53.
62. Bayly PV, Dikranian KT, Black EE, et al. Spatiotemporal evolution of apoptotic neurodegeneration following traumatic injury to the developing rat brain. Brain Res 2006;1107(1):70–81.
63. Bittigau P, Sifringer M, Pohl D, et al. Apoptotic neurodegeneration following trauma is markedly enhanced in the immature brain. Ann Neurol 1999;45(6):724–35.

64. Jacobs B, Beems T, Stulemeijer M, et al. Outcome prediction in mild traumatic brain injury: age and clinical variables are stronger predictors than CT abnormalities. J Neurotrauma 2010;27(4):655–68.
65. Santa Maria MP, Pinkston JB, Miller SR, et al. Stability of postconcussion symptomatology differs between high and low responders and by gender but not by mild head injury status. Arch Clin Neuropsychol 2001;16(2):133–40.
66. Schneider GE. Is it really better to have your brain lesion early? A revision of the "Kennard principle". Neuropsychologia 1979;17(6):557–83.
67. Pullela R, Raber J, Pfankuch T, et al. Traumatic injury to the immature brain results in progressive neuronal loss, hyperactivity and delayed cognitive impairments. Dev Neurosci 2006;28(4–5):396–409.
68. Huh JW, Widing AG, Raghupathi R. Midline brain injury in the immature rat induces sustained cognitive deficits, bihemispheric axonal injury and neurodegeneration. Exp Neurol 2008;213(1):84–92.
69. Satz P, Zaucha K, McCleary C, et al. Mild head injury in children and adolescents: a review of studies (1970–1995). Psychol Bull 1997;122(2):107–31.
70. Satz P. Mild head injury in children and adolescents. Curr Dir Psychol Sci 2001; 10:106–9.
71. Fay TB, Yeates KO, Taylor HG, et al. Cognitive reserve as a moderator of postconcussive symptoms in children with complicated and uncomplicated mild traumatic brain injury. J Int Neuropsychol Soc 2010;16(1):94–105.
72. Catale C, Marique P, Closset A, et al. Attentional and executive functioning following mild traumatic brain injury in children using the Test for Attentional Performance (TAP) battery. J Clin Exp Neuropsychol 2009;31(3):331–8.
73. Ewing-Cobbs L, Fletcher JM, Levin HS, et al. Longitudinal neuropsychological outcome in infants and preschoolers with traumatic brain injury. J Int Neuropsychol Soc 1997;3(6):581–91.
74. Dawson KS, Batchelor J, Meares S, et al. Applicability of neural reserve theory in mild traumatic brain injury. Brain Inj 2007;21(9):943–9.
75. Stern Y. What is cognitive reserve? Theory and research application of the reserve concept. J Int Neuropsychol Soc 2002;8(3):448–60.
76. Dikmen SS, Levin HS. Methodological issues in the study of mild head injury. J Head Trauma Rehabil 1993;8(3):30–7.
77. Iverson GL, Lange RT, Brooks BL, et al. "Good old days" bias following mild traumatic brain injury. Clin Neuropsychol 2010;24(1):17–37.
78. Yeates KO, Taylor HG. Neurobehavioural outcomes of mild head injury in children and adolescents. Pediatr Rehabil 2005;8(1):5–16.
79. Yeates KO. Mild traumatic brain injury and postconcussive symptoms in children and adolescents. J Int Neuropsychol Soc 2010;16(6):953–60.
80. McKinlay A, Grace RC, Horwood LJ, et al. Long-term behavioural outcomes of pre-school mild traumatic brain injury. Child Care Health Dev 2010;36(1):22–30.
81. Yeates KO, Taylor HG, Rusin J, et al. Longitudinal trajectories of postconcussive symptoms in children with mild traumatic brain injuries and their relationship to acute clinical status. Pediatrics 2009;123(3):735–43.
82. Timonen M, Miettunen J, Hakko H, et al. The association of preceding traumatic brain injury with mental disorders, alcoholism and criminality: the Northern Finland 1966 Birth Cohort Study. Psychiatry Res 2002;113(3):217–26.
83. Roncadin C, Guger S, Archibald J, et al. Working memory after mild, moderate, or severe childhood closed head injury. Dev Neuropsychol 2004; 25(1–2):21–36.

84. Ewing-Cobbs L, Barnes M, Fletcher JM, et al. Modeling of longitudinal academic achievement scores after pediatric traumatic brain injury. Dev Neuropsychol 2004;25(1–2):107–33.

85. Anderson SW, Damasio H, Tranel D, et al. Long-term sequelae of prefrontal cortex damage acquired in early childhood. Dev Neuropsychol 2000;18(3):281–96.

86. Jacobs R, Harvey AS, Anderson V. Executive function following focal frontal lobe lesions: impact of timing of lesion on outcome. Cortex 2007;43(6):792–805.

87. Catroppa C, Anderson VA, Morse SA, et al. Children's attentional skills 5 years post-TBI. J Pediatr Psychol 2007;32(3):354–69.

88. Anderson V, Catroppa C. Recovery of executive skills following paediatric traumatic brain injury (TBI): a 2 year follow-up. Brain Inj 2005;19(6):459–70.

89. McKinlay A, Dalrymple-Alford JC, Horwood LJ, et al. Long term psychosocial outcomes after mild head injury in early childhood. J Neurol Neurosurg Psychiatry 2002;73(3):281–8.

90. Anderson V, Catroppa C, Morse S, et al. Functional plasticity or vulnerability after early brain injury? Pediatrics 2005;116(6):1374–82.

91. Bonnier C, Marique P, Van Hout A, et al. Neurodevelopmental outcome after severe traumatic brain injury in very young children: role for subcortical lesions. J Child Neurol 2007;22(5):519–29.

92. Massagli TL, Fann JR, Burington BE, et al. Psychiatric illness after mild traumatic brain injury in children. Arch Phys Med Rehabil 2004;85(9):1428–34.

93. McKinlay A, Grace R, Horwood J, et al. Adolescent psychiatric symptoms following preschool childhood mild traumatic brain injury: evidence from a birth cohort. J Head Trauma Rehabil 2009;24(3):221–7.

94. Hessen E, Nestvold K, Sundet K. Neuropsychological function in a group of patients 25 years after sustaining minor head injuries as children and adolescents. Scand J Psychol 2006;47(4):245–51.

95. Hessen E, Nestvold K, Anderson V. Neuropsychological function 23 years after mild traumatic brain injury: a comparison of outcome after paediatric and adult head injuries. Brain Inj 2007;21(9):963–79.

96. Cantu RC. Recurrent athletic head injury: risks and when to retire. Clin Sports Med 2003;22(3):593–603, x.

97. Mortimer JA, van Duijn CM, Chandra V, et al. Head trauma as a risk factor for Alzheimer's disease: a collaborative re-analysis of case-control studies. EURODEM Risk Factors Research Group. Int J Epidemiol 1991;20(Suppl 2): S28–35.

98. Goldman SM, Tanner CM, Oakes D, et al. Head injury and Parkinson's disease risk in twins. Ann Neurol 2006;60(1):65–72.

99. Chen H, Richard M, Sandler DP, et al. Head injury and amyotrophic lateral sclerosis. Am J Epidemiol 2007;166(7):810–6.

100. McKee AC, Cantu RC, Nowinski CJ, et al. Chronic traumatic encephalopathy in athletes: progressive tauopathy after repetitive head injury. J Neuropathol Exp Neurol 2009;68(7):709–35.

101. McKee AC, Gavett BE, Stern RA, et al. TDP-43 proteinopathy and motor neuron disease in chronic traumatic encephalopathy. J Neuropathol Exp Neurol 2010; 69(9):918–29.

102. Fleminger S, Oliver DL, Lovestone S, et al. Head injury as a risk factor for Alzheimer's disease: the evidence 10 years on; a partial replication. J Neurol Neurosurg Psychiatry 2003;74(7):857–62.

103. Mortimer JA, French LR, Hutton JT, et al. Head injury as a risk factor for Alzheimer's disease. Neurology 1985;35(2):264–7.

104. O'Meara ES, Kukull WA, Sheppard L, et al. Head injury and risk of Alzheimer's disease by apolipoprotein E genotype. Am J Epidemiol 1997; 146(5):373–84.

105. Mehta KM, Ott A, Kalmijn S, et al. Head trauma and risk of dementia and Alzheimer's disease: The Rotterdam Study. Neurology 1999;53(9):1959–62.

106. Katzman R, Galasko DR, Saitoh T, et al. Apolipoprotein-epsilon4 and head trauma: synergistic or additive risks? Neurology 1996;46(3):889–91.

107. Mayeux R, Ottman R, Maestre G, et al. Synergistic effects of traumatic head injury and apolipoprotein-epsilon 4 in patients with Alzheimer's disease. Neurology 1995;45(3 Pt 1):555–7.

108. Plassman BL, Havlik RJ, Steffens DC, et al. Documented head injury in early adulthood and risk of Alzheimer's disease and other dementias. Neurology 2000;55(8):1158–66.

109. Gavett BE, Stern RA, Cantu RC, et al. Mild traumatic brain injury: a risk factor for neurodegeneration. Alzheimers Res Ther 2010;2(3):18.

110. Jellinger KA, Paulus W, Wrocklage C, et al. Traumatic brain injury as a risk factor for Alzheimer disease. Comparison of two retrospective autopsy cohorts with evaluation of ApoE genotype. BMC Neurol 2001;1:3.

111. Corrigan F, Pham CL, Vink R, et al. The neuroprotective domains of the amyloid precursor protein, in traumatic brain injury, are located in the two growth factor domains. Brain Res 2011;1378:137–43.

112. Smith DH, Uryu K, Saatman KE, et al. Protein accumulation in traumatic brain injury. Neuromolecular Med 2003;4(1–2):59–72.

113. Bower JH, Maraganore DM, Peterson BJ, et al. Head trauma preceding PD: a case-control study. Neurology 2003;60(10):1610–5.

114. Uryu K, Giasson BI, Longhi L, et al. Age-dependent synuclein pathology following traumatic brain injury in mice. Exp Neurol 2003;184(1):214–24.

115. Newell KL, Boyer P, Gomez-Tortosa E, et al. Alpha-synuclein immunoreactivity is present in axonal swellings in neuroaxonal dystrophy and acute traumatic brain injury. J Neuropathol Exp Neurol 1999;58(12):1263–8.

116. Gavett BE, Stern RA, McKee AC. Chronic traumatic encephalopathy: a potential late effect of sport-related concussive and subconcussive head trauma. Clin Sports Med 2011;30(1):179–88, xi.

117. Belanger HG, Spiegel E, Vanderploeg RD. Neuropsychological performance following a history of multiple self-reported concussions: a meta-analysis. J Int Neuropsychol Soc 2010;16(2):262–7.

118. Omalu BI, Bailes J, Hammers JL, et al. Chronic traumatic encephalopathy, suicides and parasuicides in professional American athletes: the role of the forensic pathologist. Am J Forensic Med Pathol 2010;31(2):130–2.

119. Guskiewicz KM, Marshall SW, Bailes J, et al. Recurrent concussion and risk of depression in retired professional football players. Med Sci Sports Exerc 2007;39(6):903–9.

120. Braak H, Braak E. Neuropathological staging of Alzheimer-related changes. Acta Neuropathol 1991;82(4):239–59.

121. Bruijn LI, Miller TM, Cleveland DW. Unraveling the mechanisms involved in motor neuron degeneration in ALS. Annu Rev Neurosci 2004;27:723–49.

122. Mulder DW, Kurland LT, Offord KP, et al. Familial adult motor neuron disease: amyotrophic lateral sclerosis. Neurology 1986;36(4):511–7.

123. Schmidt S, Kwee LC, Allen KD, et al. Association of ALS with head injury, cigarette smoking and APOE genotypes. J Neurol Sci 2010;291(1–2): 22–9.

124. Binazzi A, Belli S, Uccelli R, et al. An exploratory case-control study on spinal and bulbar forms of amyotrophic lateral sclerosis in the province of Rome. Amyotroph Lateral Scler 2009;10(5-6):361–9.

125. Armon C. Sports and trauma in amyotrophic lateral sclerosis revisited. J Neurol Sci 2007;262(1–2):45–53.

126. Dickson DW. Neuropathology of non-Alzheimer degenerative disorders. Int J Clin Exp Pathol 2009;3(1):1–23.

127. Geser F, Martinez-Lage M, Kwong LK, et al. Amyotrophic lateral sclerosis, frontotemporal dementia and beyond: the TDP-43 diseases. J Neurol 2009;256(8): 1205–14.

128. Hagel B, Meeuwisse W. Risk compensation: a "side effect" of sport injury prevention? Clin J Sport Med 2004;14:193–6.

129. Dick R, Romani WA, Agel J, et al. Descriptive epidemiology of collegiate men's lacrosse injuries: National Collegiate Athletic Association Injury Surveillance System, 1988-1989 through 2003-2004. J Athl Train 2007;42(2):255–61.

130. Crisco JJ, Fiore R, Beckwith JG, et al. Frequency and location of head impact exposures in individual collegiate football players. J Athl Train 2010;45(6): 549–59.

School and the Concussed Youth: Recommendations for Concussion Education and Management

Maegan D. Sady, PhD[a],*, Christopher G. Vaughan, PsyD[a,b,c],
Gerard A. Gioia, PhD[a,b,c]

KEYWORDS

- Concussion • Mild traumatic brain injury • Student-athlete
- Student • School • Accommodations • Management

Learning is the centerpiece of child and adolescent development. Children's organ of learning is their brain; any adverse event that impairs the brain's functioning, temporarily or permanently, poses a significant threat to learning. Traumatic brain injury (TBI) of any severity is an adverse event that can threaten the developing child's future ability to learn. Although more severe forms of TBI may be readily recognized as a threat, greater attention is being paid now to both short- and long-term effects of TBI at the milder end of the spectrum.[1] Recent advances in concussion research have provided clinicians with numerous means to recognize and assess mild TBI, commonly known as concussion. It is now widely recognized that neurometabolic

The authors have nothing to disclose.
This publication was made possible in part by CDC Award number U17/CCU323352 and grant M01RR020359 from the National Center for Research Resources (NCRR), a component of the National Institutes of Health (NIH). Other grant support included NIH number P30/HDO40677-07.
[a] Safe Concussion Outcome, Recovery & Education (SCORE) Program, Division of Pediatric Neuropsychology, Children's National Medical Center, 15245 Shady Grove Road, Suite 350, Rockville, MD 20850, USA
[b] Department of Psychiatry & Behavioral Sciences, The George Washington University School of Medicine, 2150 Pennsylvania Avenue NW, 8th Floor, Washington, DC 20037, USA
[c] Department of Pediatrics, The George Washington University School of Medicine, 2300 I Street NW, Washington, DC 20037, USA
* Corresponding author.
E-mail address: msady@childrensnational.org

Phys Med Rehabil Clin N Am 22 (2011) 701–719
doi:10.1016/j.pmr.2011.08.008
1047-9651/11/$ – see front matter © 2011 Elsevier Inc. All rights reserved.

dysfunction is a key aspect of a concussive injury, involving a cascade of neurochemical abnormalities following a force to the brain.[2] In the wake of this cascade, both physical and cognitive activity become sources of additional neurometabolic demand and stress on the brain. A basic assumption of recovery is that symptom exacerbation after physical or cognitive activity is a signal that the brain's dysfunctional neurometabolism is being pushed beyond its tolerable limits. Management of neurometabolic demands on the brain, therefore, is central to not exceeding the physiologic threshold, thus worsening symptoms and possibly prolonging recovery. Historically, physical rest has been the primary focus of attention in treatment of mild TBI. The focus on physical rest alone, however, does not address mental or cognitive exertion, which is essential for the student's functioning in school. The need for cognitive rest is advocated in the last 2 international consensus statements on concussion in sport[3,4] and requires explicit attention in the school setting. This article provides a foundation for designing a concussion education and management program in the school setting.

CONCUSSION BASICS

Mild TBI is defined as a direct or indirect force to the head that results in immediate short-lived neurologic impairment (eg, amnesia, loss of consciousness, confusion) that resolves spontaneously, typically followed by physical, cognitive, emotional symptoms and sleep disturbance.[4] Concussions result in more than 100,000 emergency department visits for children and adolescents each year,[5] with many more young people with concussion seeking treatment through physicians' offices or not at all. Timely and accurate identification and management of these injuries is especially important in children and adolescents because diagnosis rates have been increasing in high school sports.[6] Research suggests that adolescents not only are more vulnerable to brain injuries of all severity levels than adults[7] but also may take longer to recover.[8,9] There is a dearth of literature on vulnerability to brain injury and outcome in even younger youth. Increased susceptibility to concussion and its effects may be because of less-developed neck muscles for stability, hormonal influences,[10] or greater vulnerability during neural development,[11] but there is also something to be said about maturity level and the child's or adolescent's ability to follow treatment recommendations. Young individuals have multiple adults who interact with and care for them throughout each day, such as parents, teachers, guidance counselors, coaches, and athletic trainers. When there is a brain injury of any severity, these individuals must be united in their efforts to bring the young student athlete back to health and full participation in academic, sports, and recreational activities.

Physiologic Effects of Concussion

A basic understanding of the underlying physiologic effects of concussive injury to the brain is helpful in directing treatment efforts for the student in school. Acceleration and deceleration forces shake the brain inside the skull, setting off a complex cascade of shifts in ionic concentrations, release of excitatory amino acids, altered brain glucose metabolism, lactate accumulation, and reduced cerebral blood flow, along with temporary disruptions in neural membranes that, together, result in impaired connectivity, changes in neurotransmission, and a veritable energy crisis.[2,12] These neurophysiologic changes can be understood as a neurologic "software" problem rather than a "hardware" problem; current evidence suggests that concussive injuries rarely result in identifiable cell death or other structural changes.[12] When the neural software is impaired, the brain attempts to return to its normal state, temporarily forced to use a less-efficient anabolic metabolism. The clinical signs and symptoms of concussion are believed to be direct manifestations of this underlying neurometabolic cascade. Any additional activity the individual undertakes, whether physical or cognitive, becomes a source of additional neurometabolic demand on the fragile recovering brain system. If that activity becomes excessive, the cycle of inadequate metabolism and energy is perpetuated, and symptoms worsen. Indefinite prolonging of this energy crisis may have additional consequences to neuronal integrity. Therefore, activity levels must be carefully managed in students to facilitate a fast and effective recovery.

RECOVERY FROM CONCUSSION

Recovery from concussion is a process along dual continua of severity and time. Severity is multidimensional and includes not only the number and type of symptoms but also the individual's sensitivity to physical and cognitive exertion. Time can be defined in terms of early postinjury (usually the first few days) and later weeks. There are multiple preinjury and injury characteristics that have been found to influence recovery time.[13–19] Although concussion has obvious effects on learning (eg, reduced energy level, concentration, and short-term memory), there is also increasing evidence that using a concussed brain to learn can worsen concussion symptoms and perhaps even prolong recovery.[20]

Determining the end point of recovery from a concussive injury is multifaceted and includes several criteria: return of neurocognitive functioning to preinjury levels, return of balance function to preinjury levels, absence of symptoms (or return to preinjury levels) when the individual is at rest, and absence of symptoms when the individual engages in physical or cognitive activity. Each facet of recovery may resolve along a different time line. For example, some individuals report symptom resolution but continue to demonstrate cognitive impairment on neuropsychological testing[21–27] and/or ongoing metabolic abnormalities.[28,29] Recovery time is highly variable, from days to weeks to months, and is not easily predicted at the time of injury.[30] For example, some studies of high school and college athletes (mostly football players) report recovery of symptoms and neurocognitive functioning within about 7 to 10 days,[31,32] yet other studies document a substantial proportion of athletes who continue to experience symptoms and/or neurocognitive impairment well beyond this period.[30,33]

Multiple factors interact to influence recovery, including premorbid characteristics, the type of sport and/or mechanism of injury, and the age and gender of the individual. Research on predictors of prolonged recovery has been growing, and there is clear evidence that several preinjury and injury factors may prolong recovery, such as premorbid learning disability or attention-deficit/hyperactivity disorder,[13] anxiety or depression,[14–16] experience of headache,[17,18] presence of amnesia or loss of consciousness, or previous concussion.[17,19]

Effects of Concussion on Learning

Concussion has both direct and indirect, and often striking, effects on learning. The symptoms themselves can make efficient processing difficult. The physical/somatic symptoms of concussion, including headache, blurry vision, light/noise sensitivity, and fatigue, can affect a student's ability to function in the classroom. Sleep disruption during childhood and adolescence is related to cognitive, behavioral, and mood changes,[34] and sleep disturbance is not uncommon after concussion. In addition, difficulty falling asleep and increased need for sleep can make staying awake and alert in class difficult.

A relatively understudied but important phenomenon is the impact of emotional symptoms on learning after a concussion. Clinical experience indicates that anxiety can be both a direct and indirect effect of concussion, and anxiety symptoms can further impair cognitive functioning as well as interfere with students' compliance with treatment recommendations. Adolescents in particular have a tendency to try to "work through" their symptoms because the stress associated with missing class or not completing their work can seem, in the short term, more unbearable than the symptoms. In addition, experiencing prolonged recovery can lead to or exacerbate emotional symptoms (eg, frustration, anxiety, depression), which may in turn negatively affect individuals' perception of their cognitive functioning.[35]

The cognitive symptoms of concussion include feeling foggy or slowed down and difficulty concentrating or remembering. There are also measurable effects of concussion on cognitive functioning, including decreased learning and memory, decreased attention, and slowed processing speed and reaction time.[36,37]

Effects of Learning on Concussion

In addition to the cognitive symptoms that are often experienced after concussion, engaging in cognitive activity (eg, attending class, reading, studying) is hypothesized to stress the already underenergized brain, resulting in worsening of symptoms and potentially prolonged recovery.[20] The experience of worsening symptoms following cognitive activity has been referred to as the effects of cognitive exertion, although it may be more appropriately termed as the effects of cognitive over-exertion. In fact, the concept of cognitive exertion can be represented on a continuum that ranges from no activity (ie, full rest) to full activity (ie, no rest). The therapeutic goal during concussion recovery is to find an appropriate level of cognitive exertion that does not exacerbate symptoms or cause the reemergence of previously resolved symptoms.[38] It is unlikely that this goal would entail complete rest, but instead a level of cognitive activity that is below one's symptom threshold (ie, subsymptom threshold).

Cognitive overexertion is very commonly reported in clinical settings,[39] and its prevention is of utmost importance. In a group of students who sustained concussions and were treated in the authors' clinic (n = 72), more than 80% reported increased postconcussion symptoms after cognitive exertion 1 month after injury.[11] In contrast, in this sample of students, less than 40% reported an increase in symptoms with physical exertion. One factor contributing to this difference was the greater number of restrictions placed on students' physical activity (43% reported restrictions) versus their cognitive activity (only 3% reported restrictions).

The antidote to cognitive overexertion is cognitive rest, which has been identified as one of the cornerstones of concussion management[4] and involves avoiding excessive demand on neurometabolic processes associated with cognitive activities. Similar to the instructions a physician would provide to an athlete to avoid bearing weight on an injured ankle or knee to promote recovery, the concept of cognitive rest involves avoidance of mental challenges during the initial postconcussion stage. A careful balance between cognitive activity and rest is paramount in these early stages of recovery and beyond. Children and adolescents, with the help of adults involved in their care, should maintain a level of cognitive activity that does not make symptoms worse or reappear[38] to avoid exacerbating symptoms and possibly delaying recovery.[4,39,40]

The level of activity that is tolerable (ie, does not worsen or create symptoms) is unique for every individual and changes throughout the course of the recovery time line, both as time passes and symptoms resolve or change, and as the individual's sensitivity to activity changes. For example, for a highly symptomatic individual in the early stages of recovery who is sensitive to environmental stimuli (eg, noise, light), rest may mean lying in a dark quiet room. Particularly early on, cognitive rest may require a student to refrain from almost all activities that involve cognitive exertion, such as working on a computer, watching television, using a cell phone, reading, playing video games, text messaging, or listening to loud music. Some student athletes may need a full- or part-time hiatus from school while symptomatic.[4,40] For another individual further along in recovery who is less severely symptomatic and less sensitive to environmental stimuli, light reading or short periods of television or listening to music can be relaxing. One challenge in managing activities to reduce symptoms is that many student athletes have difficulty complying with instructions to limit or completely avoid cognitive activities because these activities are routine parts of their day, used to avoid boredom and to communicate with teammates and friends. For parents and other adults managing a child's activities after a concussion, prescribing and enforcing limitations require striking a careful balance between prioritizing rest while still allowing some activities in short bursts, provided these activities do not make symptoms worse.

Proactive management of activities is likely beneficial for recovery, although prospective studies of activity management and recovery have not been conducted in humans. In rats, early postinjury physical activity (within the first 2 weeks) led to lower learning and memory performance and reduction in plasticity-related proteins, whereas rats that engaged in activity later in recovery showed improved learning and memory.[41] In humans, a retrospective chart review found that higher levels of cognitive and physical activity during recovery were associated with greater neurocognitive deficits and higher symptom reports.[20]

RETURN TO ACTIVITIES FOLLOWING A CONCUSSION
Return to Cognitive Activity

Concussion management guidelines have begun to appreciate the effects of cognitive exertion on concussion symptoms and management,[3,4] and the process of academic return is gaining attention in scientific literature, the press, and legislation. Careful management of neurometabolic demands on the brain during recovery, including what is needed for cognitive activity, must avoid exceeding the threshold that produces symptom exacerbation. Children and adolescents spend most of each day engaging in cognitive activity, from classroom work and note taking to homework, and from video games to texting and social networking. Although some of these activities take place at home, many of them occur in the school environment. Thus, school personnel must play an important role in managing these cognitive activities to facilitate concussion recovery. A school with concussion policies and procedures implemented before a student sustains an injury is better prepared to manage a successful return. The basic components of a school-based concussion management plan, including who should be involved and appropriate interventions, are outlined in the following section. Although there is no plan that works for everyone, there are certain symptom and neurocognitive presentations that indicate a need for accommodations, and these are discussed in more detail in the final section of this article.

Return to Physical Activity

Students with a concussion must be restricted from physical activity, sports, and playground activity until a health care professional with expertise in concussion evaluation and management provides clearance for the student to return to play. This restriction is to first protect the student athlete from sustaining another blow to the head and already more vulnerable brain. A second blow can lead to catastrophic injury or, at the very least, significant worsening of symptoms and/or considerably prolonged recovery. Another reason for restricting activity is that physical activity can cause symptoms to worsen during the early stages of recovery. Protocols for returning to physical activity, including recess, physical education (PE) class, recreation, and sports, include graduated steps to increase activity levels while ensuring that symptoms do not worsen or return at each step before progressing to the next level.

The gradual return-to-play protocol for sports activity typically begins after complete resolution of symptoms at physical rest and no symptom return with cognitive exertion. It is essential that school and medical personnel communicate with coaches, PE teachers, and athletic trainers about the student's cognitive progress when planning a return to physical activity. Students should be able to participate in their typical academic activities, including attending full days of school and completing work without accommodations, with no return of symptoms, before return to play is considered. This provides important information about the postconcussion neurometabolic status of the student athlete's brain.

At the 2001 Vienna consensus meeting of the International Concussion in Sport Group, concussion recovery strategies focused on a graduated program of return to physical activity.[42] Athletic trainers and sports medicine physicians have been instrumental in promoting and facilitating these protocols. General guidance for having a student athlete return to sports, PE class, or recess may include transitioning the injured student from no participation to limited participation, by gradually engaging only in low-risk drills or activities or playing with increased adult supervision. The gradual return to play in sports takes place in 5 progressive steps,[42] with careful monitoring for return of any post-concussive symptoms at each stage. The first step begins with light physical activity not involving any jarring of the head (eg, walking, elliptical, or stationary bicycle) for relatively short periods. The second step involves an increase in the intensity and duration of activity, introducing movement such as jogging and sports-specific drills. The third step continues to increase the intensity and duration of physical activity incorporating movement in all 3 planes (forward-backward, side-to-side, and up-and-down). Choice of activities in each of the first 3 steps should be made with minimal risk of reinjury. The fourth step involves the athlete participating in controlled scrimmages or other supervised contact play. The final step is participation in full contact competition, where appropriate. Return to play for nonathletes, for whom a systematic plan of gradual return is not readily built in, necessitates a more creative program that might be conducted by an athletic trainer or sports physical therapist to ensure that engaging in physically challenging activities does not result in return of symptoms.

CONCUSSION PROGRAMS IN SCHOOLS

There is a need in schools across the country for widespread concussion awareness, education, and management programs. Although several states have passed legislation and implemented policies regarding education and management of athletic return to play for injured student athletes, less attention has been given to formal policies and procedures that support the recovery of the student role of the student athlete. In an attempt to address this gap in policy, legislation has been introduced in Congress by the Education and Workforce Committee that, in addition to providing return-to-play guidelines, outlines necessary education and policies needed for managing concussions' effects on learning and school participation.[43] Regardless of whether such legislation passes, structured programmatic changes in schools are needed because many are simply not prepared to assume management of students with concussion. To help the authors understand the magnitude of this need, parents of students with concussions seen recently in their clinic ($n = 49$) were asked about their child's return to school after injury. Of those surveyed, only 24% reported that they were aware of a written plan for concussion management at their child's school, and it is unknown whether these plans included academic accommodations and return to cognitive activities as opposed to return to play, the latter of which is the focus of most existing plans. Almost half of the parents (43%) were moderately or very concerned about their child's return to school, and 38% worried that their child's grades had been or would be affected after the injury. Most parents surveyed (70%) indicated that their child needed some kind of support on returning to school, with the most commonly endorsed accommodations being rest breaks and extra time for assignments and tests. Almost a quarter (23%) of parents who stated that their children need support were not sure what form that might take, highlighting the importance of including medical and academic professionals in the development of a temporary accommodation plan specific to each injured student.

There are 3 steps to designing and implementing a concussion program in a school: (1) establishing policies and procedures, (2) educating school personnel, and (3) implementing the plans for students who sustain concussions. Just as in other accommodation-based educational plans, the plan for each student with concussion requires individualization, involving the cooperation and creativity of multiple school personnel and ongoing assessment and adjustment of the plan throughout recovery. The various steps occur in a specific timeline throughout the course of the school year, with development of the policy and procedures and education conducted before the school year, review and monitoring of policies and concussions throughout the year, and active management being implemented as soon as an injury is suspected or identified. **Table 1** outlines the various processes described along this time line, with delineation of responsible parties, when various steps should be completed, and the benchmarks for completion.

Policies and Procedures

The first step in school-based concussion education and management is to develop policies and procedures to help returning students succeed as they recover from a concussion. As noted in the Centers for Disease Control's (CDC's) "Heads Up to Schools: Know Your Concussion ABCs" toolkit,[44] policy statements should include the following: (1) school's commitment to safety, (2) a brief description of concussion, (3) a plan to help students ease back into school life (learning, social activity), and (4) information on when students can safely return to physical activity after a concussion. To ensure that concussions are identified early and managed effectively, an action plan must be in place before the start of the school year based on the policies and procedures. All appropriate school and athletic staff should know about the plan and be trained to implement it.

The school policy should describe how to create and maintain safe school environments. All school staff and administrators must be encouraged to keep the physical space safe, stairs and hallways clear of clutter, rugs secured to the floor, and the surfaces of all areas where students are physically active, such as playing fields and playgrounds, safe. Additional safety considerations regarding concussion prevention can include a commitment to appropriate use of safety equipment (eg, helmets) and instruction in safe playing techniques (eg, tackling and checking approaches to reduce the chances of injury). Descriptions of concussion should be generated from scientific

Table 1
School concussion management: activities and responsibilities

Activity	Responsible Parties	Completion Date	Evidence of Completion
Before school year			
1. Concussion management policies & procedures	School administration (school nurse, counselor, psychologist)	Before start of school year	Written policy in school manual, copy provided to all school staff
2. Development of school concussion resource team	School administration, including school nurse, counselor, psychologist, designated teacher, athletic trainer	Before start of school year	Written policy in school manual
3. Examine teaching/support methods to support recovery, maximize learning/performance, and reduce symptom exacerbation	School administration, including school nurse, counselor, psychologist	Before start of school year	Written policies on teaching methods
4. Teacher/staff education & training (online video training, CDC school professional fact sheet)	Teacher, school counselor, school nurse, administrators	Before start of school year	Verification of completion provided to school administration
5. Develop list of concussion resources for education, consultation & referral (medical, school, state/local Brain Injury Association)	School administration	Before start of school year	List of resources provided in policies & procedures, available to school staff & families

During school year (preinjury)			
1. Review/reinforce concussion policy and procedures	School administration, school nurse/counselor	First faculty meeting, parent back to school night	Verbal report
2. Monitoring for injury, parent informed of injury	Coach, athletic trainer, school health personnel	Day of injury	Concussion symptom checklist, parent provided ACE Postconcussion Home/School Instructions
School management (postinjury)			
1. Medical evaluation & school treatment planning	Licensed health care professional with concussion training, school concussion resource team	Early postinjury	Plan for school return/activity
2. Gradual return to school program	Licensed health care professional with concussion training, school concussion resource team	When medically determined to tolerate >30 minutes of cognitive activity	Medical documentation
3. In-school observation, monitoring, & supports	School concussion resource team	Ongoing	Concussion symptom checklist
4. Clearance for full return to academics	Licensed health care professional with concussion training, school concussion resource team	Asymptomatic with full cognitive exertion	Medical documentation (provided to family and school)

Abbreviations: ACE, Acute Concussion Evaluation; CDC, Centers for Disease Control and Prevention.

literature, with emphasis on how to recognize concussions and their signs and symptoms.

An essential part of the plan to help students ease back into school life is to identify the key personnel and the roles each will play to support the student's return. Key team members include the school nurse/health aide, school counselor, school psychologist, speech/language pathologist, and school administrator. In addition, all school staff must understand the general principles for supporting the student's return, including classroom teachers, PE teachers, coaches, and staff who supervise free time such as lunch and recess. Supporting a student recovering from a concussion requires a collaborative approach among school professionals, health care professionals, parents, and students. School policies should specify how school personnel will be informed about a returning student's injury and specific symptoms and ways they can assist with the student's transition process and making accommodations for a student. Existing mechanisms for supporting students such as response to intervention (RTI) services or a 504 plan should be considered. An RTI approach is an active, collaborative, problem-solving approach amongst the teaching staff, student, and parents that dynamically assesses the student's needs, designs the necessary academic and/or behavioral interventions, continuously monitors the student's progress, and adjusts the interventions accordingly to meet the student's needs. Section 504 is an educational support mechanism that is implemented when students have a defined disability (temporary or permanent) that affects their academic learning and performance. The return-to-physical-activity team must be able to monitor activities, symptoms, and cognitive and balance testing or conduct consultation with professionals who have training in concussion management and the administration and interpretation of test results.

Education

The second step in developing a schoolwide or systemwide concussion management program involves educating school personnel about (1) concussions and their effects and (2) each professional's role in management when an injury occurs. Ideally, education about concussion would occur before the start of the school year so that teachers, counselors, administrators, coaches, and nurses alike are prepared to identify a concussion when it occurs. Participants should also learn about the potential long-term effects of concussion and the dangers of returning to activity too soon. The more people know about a concussion before it happens, the more likely it is that the concussion will be managed correctly from the start, reducing potential complications from returning to activities too soon. To aid in information dissemination, the CDC has published a toolkit of educational materials for school personnel[44] that parallels the materials available in the physicians' toolkit.[45] These materials highlight the symptoms and recovery course of students as they apply to the school setting and provide a starting point for concussion education.

Intervention/Management Plans

In tandem with concussion education, a schoolwide management plan should be implemented with review and updating each year before the start of the school year. A model program, developed by school and medical practitioners in Colorado, is entitled REAP (for Reduce, Educate, Accommodate, Pace) and includes structured guidelines for the role of parents, students, school academic teams, school physical activity coordinators, and medical professionals in return to both physical and cognitive activities after concussion.[46] Because no two concussions are the same, there is not a "one size fits all" plan, but there should be a team assembled with clearly defined roles. Each effective management plan must involve injured students, their parents, and a carefully coordinated team of school personnel. The members of the school team vary based on school resources but typically include some combination of the athletic trainer, guidance counselor, school nurse, all teachers, and the school psychologist or social worker as needed.[47] One person (eg, nurse or athletic trainer) should regularly track symptoms, looking for improvement or worsening, and communicate changes to the rest of the team. The student's guidance counselor or school psychologist is essential for coordinating accommodations and using the symptom log to guide adjustments.[47] In addition to self-reported symptoms, the injured student's teachers should attend to the existence of the cognitive effects of injuries: increased problems paying attention or concentrating, increased problems remembering or learning new information, needing longer to complete tasks or assignments, greater irritability and less tolerance for stressors, and an increase in symptoms (eg, headache, fatigue) when doing schoolwork.[44]

Throughout the course of recovery, it is essential that student athletes receive a consistent message from all school staff about expectations and accommodations during recovery. As soon as a student is identified as having sustained a concussion, symptoms should be assessed. The first decision must then be whether the student should or should not attend school. The model often used, in which students attempt to return for full days while still symptomatic without school personnel knowing their status, is a trial and error approach that too frequently results in error. A highly symptomatic student should be kept home to rest because it can be reasonably assumed that attempts to participate in academic activities will only worsen symptoms. Depending on symptom status, students can be sent home with some schoolwork to try in small blocks of time to help determine whether and when they are able to participate in cognitive activity. Some students return to school with specific recommendations from a concussion professional, which can be implemented according to the school's resources. If specific recommendations are not made by a concussion professional, the academic team coordinator should proactively develop a schedule with breaks and reduce the student's workload before symptoms are exacerbated. Students who are not already seeing a concussion professional for follow-up should be referred to such a professional if the student cannot manage cognitive demands or if cognitive rest does not facilitate recovery.

COMPONENTS OF A SUCCESSFUL GRADUAL RETURN TO COGNITIVE ACTIVITIES

By assessing symptoms and, when possible, neurocognitive status at the outset, proactive modifications to the school schedule can help prevent the effects of cognitive overexertion. Expectations can then be increased in a gradual, stepwise manner as symptoms allow. A systematic program of gradual return to academic demands after a concussion is important for several reasons. First, this program assures that cognitive demands are below the symptom threshold (ie, not of the duration or intensity to cause symptoms to return or increase). Second, there may be psychological benefits (eg, lowered stress) in reassuring injured students that they can handle the return to school. The concept of the gradual return applies to most, if not all, returning student athletes, but the implementation of the gradual return needs to be both individualized and able to change over time as the child recovers.[47] Some gradual returns may be quite rapid (eg, a student demonstrates ability to manage increasing amounts of studying through the weekend), whereas others will be prolonged (eg, a week or more attending only a class or two during the day). In those students with more severe symptoms and more prolonged restriction from school, a gradual return reinforces their ability to handle smaller amounts of schoolwork, thereby reducing the stress and anxiety caused by returning to academics. For a child who also sustained other physical injuries along with concussion, a partial return to school could also provide benefit to help with medication management for pain or orthopedic needs (eg, crutches, wrist splints, and so forth).

Practical Considerations

The timing and rate of return to school must be monitored carefully on an individual basis. Although a student who has already missed a prolonged period of school because of significant symptoms may need to return at a slow and gradual pace, sometimes an initial period of complete rest facilitates return to a full schedule of academics quickly. Alternatively, someone who has prematurely returned to school and kept pace with schoolwork despite active symptoms may require a longer period of restricted academics and a more gradual return to facilitate recovery.

Effective communication from medical professionals to school personnel regarding return to academic activities is important. Forceful requests may be met with resistance. However, most teachers are open to guidance, and reasonable recommendations as to how best to help the injured student return successfully will have a greater chance of successful implementation. To maximize successful return to school and minimize negative events, careful collaborative planning is important.

The primary guideline for helping a student return to school is the symptom pattern. As previously discussed, emerging or increasing symptoms are an indication of cognitive overexertion, that is, too much demand on the brain's dysfunctional metabolism. The workload or activities, therefore, should be reduced to keep symptoms from increasing. Remaining below the symptom threshold (ie, subsymptom threshold) is the therapeutic goal such that the physical or cognitive demands (or combination of the two) do not cause symptoms to return or worsen. Thus, most activities (except, of course, those with a potential risk of a re-injury) that do not cause symptoms to increase should be allowable as long as rest breaks are taken at the point when, or ideally just before, symptoms emerge or worsen. It is important to reinforce that all types of activities-cognitive, physical, emotional, and social-may bring individuals closer to their symptom threshold. This threshold is different across individuals and changes over the course of recovery. Another role, primarily for the medical professional, is to help arrange the environment in a way that allows for students to do as much "normal activity" as possible without crossing their individual symptom threshold. Some general modifications are provided in the following sections, but a careful assessment of symptoms, and creativity on the part of the clinician, is important for an individualized recovery plan.

Scheduling Considerations

When planning for the return to school, parents may test the symptom threshold at home by having children do work for set periods (eg, 15, 30, or 45 minutes) to see how long they can sustain concentration without increased symptoms. On returning to school, modifications may include abbreviated time at school, scheduled rest breaks (and/or self-initiated rest breaks with a pass to leave class whenever symptoms flare), and modified or limited coursework or tests. Different teachers approach academics and students from different perspectives, and finding classes that are most meaningful to students and teachers who are the most understanding and supportive may be the best classes for students to begin their return. This is not, however, always the case. Some teachers may be less forgiving of missed class time, and it may be better for the student to return to that setting to avoid the added stress of a potentially negative evaluation. This may also be an opportunity for school administration to educate and counsel the teacher on appropriate postinjury expectations.

Accommodations for Neurocognitive Deficits

The neurocognitive deficits associated with concussion include decreased reaction time or speed of processing, concentration problems, short-term or working memory deficits, problems with new learning and memory consolidation, and cognitive fatigue. These problems interfere with school performance and require explicit accommodations. For example, concentration or memory problems suggest the need for limited, modified, or no testing at that stage of recovery. Slowed processing speed suggests a need for additional time to complete work and review material. **Table 2** summarizes the link between neuropsychological deficits and functional school problems, with suggested accommodations.

Symptom-Specific Considerations

In addition to the general guidance for sports and academic activities, careful attention to specific symptoms and situations that may make symptoms worse is important. Individuals with different types of primary symptoms may require different accommodations, which also are summarized in **Table 2**. High levels of somatic symptoms may call for environmental adjustments. For example, a student who experiences headache onset or worsening with cognitive activity should be allowed to leave class to rest whenever needed. The school nurse should be involved in careful monitoring of headaches and pain medication use in these students because students should not return to class if the only way they can tolerate cognitive activity is to take medicine. A student who is sensitive to noise may need to avoid eating in the cafeteria during lunchtime or should consider traveling between classes outside of the usual between-class times. Children with dizziness or complaints of balance problems may need a pass to travel between classes before the usual time to avoid injury in crowded hallways. Accommodations for students who are experiencing fatigue should carefully consider scheduling. Even for students who are not displaying neurocognitive deficits, performance can decrease over time. For a student who is ready to take examinations, teachers should offer reduced or modified testing (eg, space out finals so that there is only 1 per day, administer tests in multiple short sessions, allow some portions to be completed orally).

A student's sleep-related symptoms can influence the decision of which classes to attend when schedule reduction is needed; a student who is experiencing difficulty falling asleep may be allowed to sleep in later, missing their morning classes, with the goal of returning to a normal sleep schedule over time. A student who wakes up symptom free but experiences symptom exacerbation throughout the day may find it more beneficial to attend morning classes and nap or rest in the afternoon before attempting homework.

As described earlier, the concussion itself can result in emotional symptoms (eg, worry, sadness), and the experience of neurocognitive difficulties can further exacerbate emotional difficulties. The student's emotional state needs to be taken into consideration to facilitate a smooth transition back to cognitive activities. Many students experience a decrease in stress and anxiety simply by knowing that the educational team is united and has proactively offered accommodations. Sometimes simple scheduling considerations can help reduce anxiety; for example, a student who is anxious about missing classes may find it helpful to rotate which classes they attend each day in order to attend each subject a few times each week. Students who report

Table 2
Accommodations for postconcussion effects affecting school

Postconcussion Effect	Functional School Problem	Accommodation/ Management Strategy
Neuropsychological deficits		
Attention/concentration	Short focus on lecture, classwork, homework	Shorter assignments, break down tasks, lighter work load
Working memory	Holding instructions in mind, reading comprehension, mathematics calculation, writing	Repetition, written instructions, use of calculator, shorter reading passages
Memory consolidation/ retrieval	Retaining new information, accessing learned information when needed	Smaller chunks to learn, recognition cues
Processing speed	Keep pace with work demand, process verbal information effectively	Extended time, slow down verbal information, comprehension checking
Fatigue	Decreased arousal/activation to engage basic attention, working memory	Rest breaks during classes, homework, and examinations
Symptoms		
Headaches	Interferes with concentration	Rest breaks
Light/noise sensitivity	Symptoms worsen in bright or loud environments	Wear sunglasses, seating away from bright sunlight or other light. Avoid noisy/crowded environments such as lunchroom, assemblies, and hallways
Dizziness/balance problems	Unsteadiness when walking	Elevator pass, class transition before bell
Sleep disturbance	Decreased arousal, shifted sleep schedule	Later start time, shortened day
Anxiety	Can interfere with concentration, student may push through symptoms to prevent falling behind	Reassurance from teachers and team about accommodations, workload reduction, alternate forms of testing
Depression/withdrawal	Withdrawal from school or friends because of stigma or activity restrictions	Time built in for socialization
Cognitive symptoms	Concentrating, learning	See specific cognitive accommodations (above)
Symptom sensitivity	Symptoms worsen with overactivity, resulting in any of the earlier-mentioned problems	Reduce cognitive or physical demands below symptom threshold, provide rest breaks, complete work in small increments until symptom threshold increases

emotional symptoms throughout their recovery need support and guidance from their guidance counselor, school psychologist, and/or a private therapist.

Perhaps the most obvious symptoms necessitating school accommodations are those that are cognitive in nature. In general, many accommodations typically provided for students with other learning and attentional problems may be appropriate temporary accommodations for students recovering from concussion. Students experiencing decreased concentration and memory capacity should be provided with lecture outlines or another student's notes to ease the burden of simultaneous listening and writing. Other accommodations to consider include allowing flexibility in assignment deadlines and postponing tests (particularly high stakes, such as final examinations and Scholastic Aptitude Tests). Time extensions and rescheduling should be weighed carefully against the future burden of a large amount of makeup work. Students who have finally returned to their baseline symptoms and cognitive functioning may regress in their recovery or experience unnecessary stress if faced with this burden. Especially for younger student athletes and those with relatively short recovery times (1–2 weeks), teachers should consider excusing all assignments during acute phase and basing grades on work completed before injury and after recovery. Extra tutoring may be helpful for students who have missed a lot of class time, but, again, caution should be used because facilitating exposure to learning in these ways may increase cognitive demands and cause increased neurometabolic strain. Careful monitoring should be used.

Precautions

The gradual return is not without its challenges. Students who are once again given permission to return to academics in any capacity may take the opportunity to overdo physical and mental activities, despite prescribed restrictions, thus putting them at risk for prolonging their recovery. Students who are present in school may also have a large amount of demands placed on them by well-intentioned teachers who see the presence of the student (and an absence of any external signs of injury) as an indication that they are capable of completing all of their work. Symptoms and neuropsychological deficits can resolve at different times for different people, so teachers should be aware that students who report being symptom free may not yet be able to perform fully at preinjury levels or successfully return to their full workload and schedule. In addition, well-meaning teachers may not appreciate the full scope of the cumulative demands placed on the student athletes by all their teachers. Well-coordinated efforts by school personnel, such as the guidance counselor or school psychologist, can help avoid this problem. A student who is at school and therefore seems available to begin completing makeup work may be asked to stay after school or receive extra tutoring to catch up on assignments. Again, careful coordination among teachers and guidance staff is the best way to avoid these unnecessary burdens.

SUMMARY

Concussions are gaining increased awareness in schools, sports, media, and research, and both personal experience and research data support the fact that these injuries can have a significant impact, at least temporarily, on a child's or adolescent's participation in school, social activities, and sports/recreational activities. A concussive injury is a direct or indirect blow to the head that results in a neurometabolic cascade and ensuing cellular energy crisis in the brain, leaving the brain vulnerable to additional injury during the recovery phase. The ensuing symptoms and neurocognitive effects of concussion affect learning and performance, and many students engaging in cognitive activity shortly after a concussion experience symptom exacerbation and increased difficulty with work completion, concentrating, and remembering. Students who are highly symptomatic and try to maintain full academic schedules quickly realize that they will need temporary accommodations to prevent falling behind and effects on their grades.

Athletic return-to-play protocols have been a focus of concussion management for quite awhile, with an emphasis on gradual return to physical activities so that reinjury does not occur before full recovery. Legislation regarding the implementation of these protocols has been passed in a growing number of states, making the transition back to sports and recreation both safer and more predictable. In contrast, protocols for return to cognitive activity in school setting are only beginning to gain momentum, and current legislation typically has not included provisions for this process. Whether or not protocols for return to academics are mandated by legislation, to support the recovery and academic needs of the recovering student, systematic efforts must be initiated as soon as possible.

Successful gradual return to cognitive activities requires coordination among school personnel who are educated about the effects of concussions on students and are committed to providing accommodations for the symptoms and neurocognitive deficits that result, continuously monitoring symptoms, and adjusting interventions accordingly until recovery. Team members include a range of school personnel, such as guidance counselor, nurse/health aide, school psychologist, teachers, PE and coaching staff, and athletic trainers, as well as the student, parents, and treating medical professionals. Key personnel would implement a well-developed accommodations plan that is specific to the recovering student's needs as soon as the concussion is suspected or identified. Scheduling and other symptom-specific accommodations would be proactively introduced to reduce the secondary effects of cognitive overexertion. A secondary focus of the plan for professionals could be to coordinate efforts to reduce the student's academic and emotional burden to facilitate recovery. The guidelines presented in this article can assist a school system in the development of its policies and procedures and also help the treating medical professional design a school-sensitive individualized plan.

The benefits of active management of cognitive and physical activities are numerous. Well-supported students can focus on resting and recovering without having to spend excess energy on trying to keep up with their academic workload, fighting for accommodations, or becoming anxious about whether their grades will suffer. Although future research is needed, it is possible that proactive management could reduce recovery times by ensuring less cognitive overexertion and stress, and therefore less misguided energy away from neurometabolic recovery. Involving school personnel in the active and continuous monitoring of cognitive activities and symptoms provides a better determination of symptom resolution both at rest and with cognitive activity. As a secondary benefit, continuous monitoring and active cognitive support can result in safer and possibly speedier recovery, providing important data to assist the decision about when to initiate the athlete's gradual return to sports participation.

REFERENCES

1. Kirkwood MW, Yeates KO, Taylor HG, et al. Management of pediatric mild traumatic brain injury: a neuropsychological review from injury through recovery. Clin Neuropsychol 2008;22(5):769–800.
2. Giza CC, Hovda DA. The neurometabolic cascade of concussion. J Athl Train 2001;36(3):228–35.
3. McCrory P, Matser E, Cantu R, et al. Sports neurology. Lancet Neurol 2004;3(7): 435–40.

4. McCrory P, Meeuwisse W, Johnston K, et al. Consensus statement on Concussion in Sport 3rd International Conference on Concussion in Sport held in Zurich, November 2008. Phys Sportsmed 2009;37(2):141–59.
5. Bakhos LL, Lockhart GR, Myers R, et al. Emergency department visits for concussion in young child athletes. Pediatrics 2010;126(3):e550–5.
6. Lincoln AE, Caswell SV, Almquist JL, et al. Trends in concussion incidence in high school sports: a prospective 11-year study. Am J Sports Med 2011. Available at: http://www.ncbi.nlm.nih.gov.ezproxyhost.library.tmc.edu/pubmed/21278427. Accessed March 21, 2011.
7. Anderson V, Moore C. Age at injury as a predictor of outcome following pediatric head injury: a longitudinal perspective. Child Neuropsychol 1995;1(3):187.
8. Field M, Collins MW, Lovell MR, et al. Does age play a role in recovery from sports-related concussion? A comparison of high school and collegiate athletes. J Pediatr 2003;142(5):546–53.
9. Pellman EJ, Lovell MR, Viano DC, et al. Concussion in professional football: recovery of NFL and high school athletes assessed by computerized neuropsychological testing—part 12. Neurosurgery 2006;58(2):263–74 [discussion: 263–74].
10. Dick RW. Is there a gender difference in concussion incidence and outcomes? Br J Sports Med 2009;43(Suppl 1):i46–50.
11. Gioia G, Vaughan C, Reesman J, et al. Characterizing post-concussion exertional effects in the child and adolescent. J Int Neuropsychol Soc 2010;16(S1):178.
12. Barkhoudarian G, Hovda DA, Giza CC. The molecular pathophysiology of concussive brain injury. Clin Sports Med 2011;30(1):33–48, vii–iii.
13. Collins MW, Grindel SH, Lovell MR, et al. Relationship between concussion and neuropsychological performance in college football players. JAMA 1999; 282(10):964–70.
14. Mather FJ, Tate RL, Hannan TJ. Post-traumatic stress disorder in children following road traffic accidents: a comparison of those with and without mild traumatic brain injury. Brain Inj 2003;17(12):1077–87.
15. Mooney G, Speed J, Sheppard S. Factors related to recovery after mild traumatic brain injury. Brain Inj 2005;19(12):975–87.
16. Moore EL, Terryberry-Spohr L, Hope DA. Mild traumatic brain injury and anxiety sequelae: a review of the literature. Brain Inj 2006;20(2):117–32.
17. Collins MW, Field M, Lovell MR, et al. Relationship between postconcussion headache and neuropsychological test performance in high school athletes. Am J Sports Med 2003;31(2):168–73.
18. Mihalik JP, Stump JE, Collins MW, et al. Posttraumatic migraine characteristics in athletes following sports-related concussion. J Neurosurg 2005;102(5):850–5.
19. Guskiewicz KM, McCrea M, Marshall SW, et al. Cumulative effects associated with recurrent concussion in collegiate football players: the NCAA Concussion Study. JAMA 2003;290(19):2549–55.
20. Majerske CW, Mihalik JP, Ren D, et al. Concussion in sports: postconcussive activity levels, symptoms, and neurocognitive performance. J Athl Train 2008; 43(3):265–74.
21. Broglio SP, Macciocchi SN, Ferrara MS. Neurocognitive performance of concussed athletes when symptom free. J Athl Train 2007;42(4):504–8.
22. Covassin T, Elbin RJ, Nakayama Y. Tracking neurocognitive performance following concussion in high school athletes. Phys Sportsmed 2010;38(4):87–93.
23. Fazio VC, Lovell MR, Pardini JE, et al. The relation between post concussion symptoms and neurocognitive performance in concussed athletes. NeuroRehabilitation 2007;22(3):207–16.

24. Lovell MR, Collins MW, Iverson GL, et al. Recovery from mild concussion in high school athletes. J Neurosurg 2003;98(2):296–301.
25. Meehan WP, d'Hemecourt P, Comstock RD. High school concussions in the 2008-2009 academic year: mechanism, symptoms, and management. Am J Sports Med 2010;38(12):2405–9.
26. Peterson CL, Ferrara MS, Mrazik M, et al. Evaluation of neuropsychological domain scores and postural stability following cerebral concussion in sports. Clin J Sport Med 2003;13(4):230–7.
27. Van Kampen DA, Lovell MR, Pardini JE, et al. The "value added" of neurocognitive testing after sports-related concussion. Am J Sports Med 2006;34(10):1630–5.
28. Vagnozzi R, Signoretti S, Cristofori L, et al. Assessment of metabolic brain damage and recovery following mild traumatic brain injury: a multicentre, proton magnetic resonance spectroscopic study in concussed patients. Brain 2010; 133(11):3232–42.
29. Vagnozzi R, Signoretti S, Tavazzi B, et al. Temporal window of metabolic brain vulnerability to concussion: a pilot 1H-magnetic resonance spectroscopic study in concussed athletes—part III. Neurosurgery 2008;62(6):1286–95 [discussion: 1295–6].
30. McClincy MP, Lovell MR, Pardini J, et al. Recovery from sports concussion in high school and collegiate athletes. Brain Inj 2006;20(1):33–9.
31. McCrea M, Guskiewicz KM, Marshall SW, et al. Acute effects and recovery time following concussion in collegiate football players: the NCAA Concussion Study. JAMA 2003;290(19):2556–63.
32. Sim A, Terryberry-Spohr L, Wilson KR. Prolonged recovery of memory functioning after mild traumatic brain injury in adolescent athletes. J Neurosurg 2008;108(3): 511–6.
33. Collins M, Lovell MR, Iverson GL, et al. Examining concussion rates and return to play in high school football players wearing newer helmet technology: a three-year prospective cohort study. Neurosurgery 2006;58(2):275–86 [discussion: 275–86].
34. O'Brien LM. The neurocognitive effects of sleep disruption in children and adolescents. Child Adolesc Psychiatr Clin N Am 2009;18(4):813–23.
35. Reddy C, Collins M, Gioia G. Adolescent sports concussion. Phys Med Rehabil Clin N Am 2008;19(2):247–69.
36. Belanger HG, Vanderploeg RD. The neuropsychological impact of sports-related concussion: a meta-analysis. J Int Neuropsychol Soc 2005;11(4):345–57.
37. Broglio SP, Puetz TW. The effect of sport concussion on neurocognitive function, self-report symptoms and postural control: a meta-analysis. Sports Med 2008; 38(1):53–67.
38. Valovich McLeod T, Gioia G. Cognitive rest: the often neglected aspect of concussion management. Athl Ther Today 2010;15(2):1–3.
39. Logan K. Cognitive rest means I can't do what? Athletic Training & Sports Health Care 2009;1(6):251–2.
40. Purcell L. What are the most appropriate return-to-play guidelines for concussed child athletes? Br J Sports Med 2009;43(Suppl 1):i51–5.
41. Griesbach GS, Gomez-Pinilla F, Hovda DA. The upregulation of plasticity-related proteins following TBI is disrupted with acute voluntary exercise. Brain Res 2004; 1016(2):154–62.
42. Aubry M, Cantu R, Dvorak J, et al. Summary and agreement statement of the First International Conference on Concussion in Sport, Vienna 2001. Recommendations for the improvement of safety and health of athletes who may suffer concussive injuries. Br J Sports Med 2002;36(1):6–10.

43. H.R. 469. Protecting Student Athletes from Concussions Act of 2011. 2011. Available at: http://www.govtrack.us/congress/bill.xpd?bill=h112-469. Accessed May 1, 2011.
44. Centers for Disease Control. Heads up to schools: know your concussion ABCs. Atlanta (GA): Centers for Disease Control; 2010. Available at: http://www.cdc.gov/concussion/HeadsUp/schools.html#2. Accessed May 1, 2011.
45. Centers for Disease Control. Heads up: brain injury in your practice. Atlanta (GA): Centers for Disease Control; 2007. Available at: http://www.cdc.gov/concussion/headsup/physicians_tool_kit.html. Accessed May 1, 2011.
46. McAvoy K. REAP the benefits of good concussion management. Centennial (CO): Rocky Mountain Youth Sports Medicine Institute; 2010. Available at: http://rockymountainhospitalforchildren.com/sports-medicine/concussion-management/reap-guidelines.htm. Accessed May 1, 2011.
47. McGrath N. Supporting the student-athlete's return to the classroom after a sport-related concussion. J Athl Train 2010;45(5):492–8.

Youth Sports and Concussions: Preventing Preventable Brain Injuries. One Client, One Cause, and A New Law

Richard H. Adler, JD[a,b,*]

KEYWORDS

• Youth • Sports • Concussion • Brain

On Thursday October 12, 2006, 13-year-old Zackery Lystedt, like many youth athletes, had just finished his school day and was continuing with after-school sports. Zack was a good student with a 3.5 grade point average and was also considered an outstanding athlete. He played many sports and was participating on his school's football team, just south of Seattle, Washington. On this day, Zack and his team traveled to a nearby middle school for a game.

Zack was the fullback on offense, and played outside linebacker on defense. The fateful play was at the end of the first half of the game with Zack in his linebacker role. The opposing team handed the ball to its fullback who cut to the sidelines (away from Zack's position) and began heading down the sidelines toward the end zone. Zack sprinted diagonally across the field and caught up to this player at the goal line. He leaped, lunged, and tackled the player. In the process, Zack's airborne body rotated and he landed with the back of his helmet hitting the ground. When the dust cleared, as captured by sideline parent-video, Zack remained on his back in the end zone holding his helmet with both hands. He was moving his legs slowly, but he did not lose consciousness. A referee called a time-out. Per league rules at that time, Zack was required to sit out only for the next play. Zack was able to walk off the field on his own with the coach by his side. He was kept out for the next 2 plays,

[a] Adler Giersch, P.S., 300 Taylor Avenue North, Seattle, WA 98109, USA
[b] Brain Injury Association of Washington, 401 Broadway, Patricia Steel Building – 4th Floor, Seattle, WA 98122, USA
* Adler Giersch, P.S., 300 Taylor Avenue North, Seattle, WA 98109.
E-mail address: radler@adlergiersch.com

Phys Med Rehabil Clin N Am 22 (2011) 721–728
doi:10.1016/j.pmr.2011.08.010
1047-9651/11/$ – see front matter © 2011 Elsevier Inc. All rights reserved.

and then it was halftime. Zack played most of the third and fourth quarters, taking hits on offense and defense. Despite his teammates (but not his coaches) noting changes to his usual play and behavior on the field, he continued to play and was credited with scoring the go-ahead touchdown for his team as well as causing a fumble against the opposing team attempting a come-from-behind score late in the game. There were no health care professionals on the sidelines to assess Zack's condition.

At the end of the game, and after handshakes and high fives across the 50-yard line, Zack began walking off the field with his father next to him. His world then went dark. He screamed to his father that he could not see and about the searing pain in his head. He collapsed on the field in his father's arms and was airlifted to Harborview Medical Center, a Trauma I hospital in Seattle, Washington, where he underwent emergency brain surgery. Immediately following surgery, Zack developed recurrent cerebral hemorrhage and was returned to the operating room to complete bilateral craniotomies and decompressions. He was in a coma for approximately 1 month. He was not able to move any limb or even blink for a period of 9 months. He was fed via percutaneous gastrostomy for 20 months.

October 2011 marks the fifth anniversary of Zack's traumatic brain injury and his premature return to play following a mild traumatic brain injury. His life and the lives of his parents will never be the same. However, his strength of character, determination toward wellness, and sense of humor inspire all those around him. Zack's injury propelled me, his legal team, community leaders, organizations, and the state of Washington into action to prevent future preventable brain injuries in youth sports.

How did this event move from tragedy to legislative action? What remains to be done to protect youth sports participants? These issues and others are discussed in this article.

SCOPE OF THE PROBLEM AND URGENCY OF THE PUBLIC HEALTH RESPONSE

Concussions are one of the most commonly reported injuries in children and adolescents who participate in sports and recreational activities. Children and teens are among those at greatest risk for concussion. Most sports-related and recreation-related concussions seen in emergency departments each year (65%) occur among youth aged 5 to 18 years.[1] More than 38 million boys and girls, aged 5 to 18 years, participate in organized youth sports in the United States. Concussions can occur in any organized or unorganized sport or recreational activity. Although youth sports concussions often are associated with football, the rate of concussion in girl's high school soccer is almost as high. Concussions are likely inevitable in youth sports (see the article by Jinjugi elsewhere in this issue for more details). Although many of these injuries are considered mild, they can result in more serious impacts on a young developing brain and can result in functional impairment with thinking, memory, emotional, or behavioral changes. The wider community must decide whether to accept the risk that comes from an ill-informed understanding of the consequences of the premature return to practice or competition following a concussion. However, the issue of accepting the risks and consequences of traumatic brain injury in youth sports assumes that school administrators, coaches, parents, and student athletes are properly educated and informed. In Zack's situation, no one was informed, risks were taken unnecessarily, and with catastrophic consequences resulted.

The world of youth sports is large, diverse, and decentralized. Most coaches in youth sport programs are volunteers (either parents or other interested persons) who have minimal or no training in coaching or injury identification or management (including concussion), and are often juggling many commitments including full-time jobs and families.[2] Youth sports coaches are on the front line to identify and respond to concussions. They play an important role in sharing safety and injury-prevention information with athletes and parents. However, who is training the school administrators, athletic directors, coaches, the parents, and the youth athletes? Who is training the sport organization's board of directors, leaders, and managers?

A youth player must be removed from any sport following concussion because a brain injury is more dangerous than a knee injury. No one has died or been catastrophically injured from the premature return-to-play decision regarding the knee, ankle, or shoulder. An injury above the chin must be treated differently and more cautiously. But why has it been difficult to have this message absorbed, taken seriously, and adopted by all?

In Zackery Lystedt's situation, there existed a vacuum of knowledge in which tragedy filled the void.

A NEW PATH TO CONCUSSION PREVENTION AND MANAGEMENT: EDUCATION AND LEGISLATION

Effective concussion prevention requires both education and legislation. Both are embodied in the first-in-the-nation law from the state of Washington, more commonly referred to as the Zackery Lystedt Law, which is serving as the prototype and model for other states' efforts to protect youth athletes. The process and participants involved, and the barriers encountered in implementing this 2-pronged approach to concussion prevention, are described in this article.

EDUCATION: GETTING THE WORD OUT
Champions

Any effort to change the culture of acceptance surrounding concussions requires a champion to challenge current thinking and reach out to aligned organizations and key individuals to engage in meaningful dialog. My advocacy started with an educational push on youth sports concussion through the Brain Injury Association of Washington (BIA-WA), and my colleagues who are clinicians and researchers at the University of Washington. Initial educational attempts focused on the BIA-WA Web site, newsletter, social media sites, and media releases that focused on a few clear messages.

MESSAGES

1. Athletes who have concussions are at an increased risk for future concussions.
2. Repeat concussions occur before the brain has time to heal from the first one, and this often occurs within a short period of time.
3. Concussions can slow recovery or increase the likelihood of long-term problems.
4. Repeat concussions can be fatal.
5. Young people take more time to heal than adults.
6. Athletes should never play with concussion symptoms (one study of high school and college football players showed that, among those who died or were seriously impaired by a head trauma, 40% were playing with symptoms from an early concussion).
7. Concussions can affect school performance because they cause difficulty in concentrating or remembering.
8. The only remedy for concussion is rest.
9. Proper recognition and proper response to concussions when they first occur can prevent further injury or even death and can help young people perform better in school.

The organizational partnership started between BIA-WA and the Centers for Disease Control (CDC), who began the production of educational materials for use on a national basis.

THE MESSENGERS
The Lystedt Family

Although professional and advocacy groups were able to provide information and recommendations based on CDC guidelines, capturing the attention of the media and the larger community required a real-life example to coalesce energy and purpose. In 2008, the Lystedt family, after Zack's initial recovery from coma and completion of his inpatient rehabilitation, elected to share their experience and struggles in supporting Zack in his recovery to garner community interest in the prevention of sports brain injuries.

Professional Sports Teams

Another early key member of the coalition was the Seattle Seahawks organization, who learned of Zack's story from their team physician and from a meeting I had with its Chief Executive Officer and President at the time. The organization agreed to become a sponsor of the educational program being formulated by the CDC and the BIA-WA. The Seahawks were instrumental in covering the expenses and providing the human resources to launch a statewide mailing campaign. So began the educational push by delivering posters and clipboards to every coach in the state of Washington. This mailing also included a personalized letter on Seattle Seahawks stationary from the head coach at the time, Mike Holmgren, encouraging coaches to place the posters in a visible location for their athletes to see and to become more aware of the risks and consequences of concussions for youth athletes.

Media and Presentations

The next step in the educational initiative was the involvement of celebrity spokespersons. Brock Huard, former Seahawks and University of Washington quarterback and sports media figure, and Steve Raible, former Seahawks player, currently the Seahawks radio announcer, and anchor of a television news program joined the educational effort. News stories on the topic resulted and in-person presentations to athletes, parents, coaches, school administrators, and health care providers were given.

LEGISLATION: MAKING THE WORD LAW

Despite outstanding educational materials provided by the CDC, presentations provided at every level of youth sports coaching, and support by professional sports organization and media figures, reports continued of devastating brain injuries sustained by young athletes during school games or other competitive venues. My analysis of these situations led to an understanding of the limitations of an educational only campaign. First, there was an 'inconsistency gap'. Coaches of youth sports from different school districts and coaches of different sports in the same school district had varied levels of understanding and perception of concussion and its seriousness. Secondly, there was a 'stickiness problem'. For example, assume that coach A understands and implements a best-practices protocol of removing youth athletes from practice or competition and not returning them without written medical clearance. Now assume that this same coach takes a different coaching position in a different school district or even a different state. When coach A leaves the school, the concussion protocol program under that coach's direction and supervision disappears. Although general guidelines may have been recommended by the school or member association, but the coach's protocol was often a personal decision to follow best practices. Because it was not district-wide or organizationally required, it was never institutionalized into the culture of the school, its people, or the sport. There was no stickiness to concussion prevention and management. The inconsistency gap and stickiness problem combined to create a patch-quilt of varying standards from one school district to the next and even different protocols from one coach to the next within the same school district. As a result, we learned that, despite best intentions, efforts, resources, and accessibility to no-cost high-quality information, education alone does not change behavior and that more was needed to prevent preventable brain injuries in youth sports.

This realization demanded a move from the grassroots efforts that had propelled the growing community coalition into exploring a top-down approach to ensuring that consistent practices for the prevention and management of concussion in youth sports were honored. We were ready to propose legislation, and that level of commitment demanded continuation of community networking among leaders and organizations to expand the coalition.

Lobbyists and Legislators

To move into the legislative realm, a knowledgeable guide to the legislative process was invaluable. BIA-WA Board Members raised funds and engaged a knowledgeable and experienced lobbyist for this effort who helped to outline the next steps toward lawmaking: merging all the members of the coalition to create a clear message and a single voice, identifying legislative champions, and presenting the legislative argument to a broad range of state legislators. Partnering with the right lobbyist was particularly important and a decision that was made carefully and strategically; a lobbyist that is too closely associated with any single political cause is off-putting to legislators. Our lobbyist was experienced in the health care arena and had lines of communication with many legislators of both major political parties with whom we needed to work. The Lystedt family became instrumental in presenting their story, first to their own legislative representative, then to other key representatives. Our coalition continued to grow in size and political will, one key organization at a time. Groups including the Washington State Athletic Trainers Association, the Washington State Interscholastic Activities Association (WIAA), Canfield (insurance risk pool managers), Harborview Medical Center, University of Washington Medical Center, Seattle Children's Hospital, Washington State Youth Soccer Association, and the American Academy of Pediatricians (Washington Chapter), met frequently with me and others from the BIA-WA, honed its messages, and selected the spokesperson for each organization.

In the legislative process, bills are introduced and then assigned to committees that preside over the subject matter of the proposed legislation. There can be different committees hearing the same legislation (eg, health, schools, fiscal) to filter out and tinker with the language of the legislation before recommending voting (or not) on proposed legislation for the respective House and Senate chambers. If a bill is stopped in any committee in either the House or Senate side, then it is likely going 'to die' in committee and never come up for vote. From January to May 2009, keeping the bill alive was a daily effort. Our presentations were well received in each committee hearing, likely because of the simple and clear message, as well as the strong and diverse coalition of supporters including advocacy groups, youth sport organization groups, insurance risk pool groups, athletic trainers, and physicians.

The proposed legislation passed the House Education Committee unanimously and then the Senate Committee. When the legislation went to the House for vote, it was passed by a vote of 98 to 0 with Zackery and his father on the House floor to witness the historic occasion. In the Senate, it was also unanimous. The vote was 45 to 0. It was a great day for children, their brains, and sports.

CORE ELEMENTS OF THE ZACKERY LYSTEDT LAW

Key provisions of the new law require:

- Youth athletes who are 'suspected of a concussion' or head injury must be removed from practice or competition at the time of the suspected injury. In other words, "when in doubt, sit them out."
- School districts are to work with the WIAA to develop information and policies on educating coaches, youth athletes, and parents about the nature and risk of concussion, including the dangers of returning to practice or competition after a concussion or head injury.
- All student athletes and their parents/guardians must sign an information sheet about concussion and head injury before the youth athlete's initiating practice at the start of each season and for each sport.
- Youth athletes who have been removed from play must receive written medical clearance before returning to play from a licensed health care provider trained in the evaluation and management of concussion.
- Private, nonprofit youth sports associations wanting to use publicly owned play-fields must comply with this law.

THE COST OF IMPLEMENTING A CONCUSSION PREVENTION LAW

An often-asked question in moving the Lystedt legislation through the Washington House and Senate Chambers involved the cost of implementing this type of legislation. This legislation is 'revenue neutral,' meaning that it would not cost any additional funds from any state, county, local agency, or school district to implement the law. There is no mandate in our legislative language or any requirement that resources get expended to hire trained health care professions to be on the sidelines or to purchase any equipment. Those decisions are left to the sporting organization or school district involved, but they are not required. Abundant educational information was available free of charge for coaches, parents, athletes, and school professionals at the CDC Web site at www.cdc.gov/concussion and the BIA-WA Web site at www.braininjurwa.org.

ARE THERE PENALTIES IF THE LYSTEDT LAW IS VIOLATED?

In drafting the Lystedt Law, we intentionally did not embed specific consequences against a coach, team, school district, or organization into the legislation. We did not seek to have civil or criminal penalties in state law. Itemizing penalties would have been a divisive issue for different coalition partners. The legislation was framed around the core principles of education and prevention and we worked hard to keep the legislation simple. Also, in the state of Washington, as in many other states, there is an organization empowered with rule making and decision making for youth sports: the WIAA. Any rules concerning penalties in deciding how to monitor and enforce the provisions of this law should come from this organization and not the legislature. This organization already had the mandate and authority to implement and enforce rules.

THE PERCEIVED DISPARITY IN ACCESS TO QUALIFIED HEALTH CARE PROVIDERS BETWEEN RURAL AND URBAN AREAS

We also needed to carefully think through the disparity in access to health care professionals between urban and rural areas. When youth athletes were removed from practice or a game following a concussion, they would need to be medically cleared before returning. To address this concern, we made certain that the Lystedt Law did not call out a specifically licensed health care provider to participate in every evaluation on return to play. We appreciated the political need and reality that there may not be sufficient knowledgeable, accessible, and/or affordable medical specialists in rural areas to clear a youth athlete to return to play. As a result, it was important to have many types of qualified health care providers in the mix. Our legislation required that the youth athlete be cleared by a "licensed health care provider trained in the evaluation and management of concussion" and did not specify a specific type of medical specialist to provide the evaluation and clearance.

In Washington State, it was the WIAA, in its role as the sport's rule-making body for student athletes, who decided that those licensed health care providers qualified to make the return-to-play decisions included five groups: medical doctors, doctors of osteopathic medicine, physician assistants, nurse practitioners, and licensed and certified athletic trainers. (In some states, athletic trainers are certified from coursework. In Washington, athletic trainers must be certified as well as licensed by a regulatory agency with disciplinary authority.) By having a wider range of health care professionals qualified to make this evaluation, the access issue was appropriately addressed for our coalition partners and those legislators representing rural communities in our state.

CASCADING THE LYSTEDT LAW INTO PRIVATE YOUTH SPORTS ORGANIZATIONS

Laws that are promulgated by state legislative bodies cover public-supported sports organizations including athletics in public schools. However, one of the challenges was to extend the Lystedt Law to those youth athletes in private schools who were not members of the WIAA as well as in private leagues. We were stymied initially because the Lystedt Law would not extend to these organizations. Private sports organizations such as youth soccer, baseball, and lacrosse often used public lands for their practices or games. Moreover, teams from private schools often had cross-divisional scrimmages or games with public school teams, and playoff games are often held at larger venues that include public fields. Whenever a private organization or private school uses public lands, they were required to obtain and present an insurance policy indemnifying the public land owner from any potential claim of negligence during the course of the use of the public land. As a result, to extend the reach of the Lystedt Law to the private schools who are not members of the WIAA and youth sports leagues using public lands, we proposed amending the existing insurance-based mandate to also include the requirement that these organizations comply with the policies on the management of concussion and head injuries in youth sports, as per the Lystedt Law.

EARLY ANECDOTAL DATA: EDUCATION AND LEGISLATION WORKS

In Washington State, one of the major insurance risk pools for schools in Washington reported that, in 2010, 1 year following the signing of the Lystedt Law, there were no reports of death or subdural hematoma requiring surgery in any youth athlete following a football game in the entire season, and this is the first time that this has occurred in every consecutive week of boys' football in 5 years.

THE NATIONAL PUSH TO PREVENT PREVENTABLE BRAIN INJURIES FOR EVERY CHILD IN EVERY STATE

Since the enactment of the Lystedt Law, national groups have joined forces to call for the implementation of the Lystedt Law in all states throughout the United States. Key national coalition partners led by the American College of Sports Medicine (ACSM) and the National Football League (NFL) have joined BIA-WA and its coalition partners and greatly expanded our reach. Joining BIA-WA, ACSM and the NFL have been USA Football and the national governing bodies of many other youth sports organizations, National School Boards Association, National Association of School of Nurses, National Counsel of Youth Sports, National Disability Rights Network, National Athletic Trainers Association, National Association of Health and Fitness, American Academy of Physical Medicine and Rehabilitation, numerous state chapters of the Brain Injury Association of America, the American Academy of Neurology, the National Collegiate Athletic Association, and many others.

The Lystedt Law was signed by Governor Christine Gregoire on May 9, 2009, with an implementation date of July 26, 2009. Since that time, and as of the writing of this article, other states have followed Washington's initiative, including Alabama, Alaska, Arizona, Colorado, Connecticut, Delaware, Illinois, Indiana, Iowa, Kansas, Louisiana, Maryland, Massachusetts, Minnesota, Missouri, Nebraska, New Jersey, New Mexico, North Carolina, North Dakota, Oklahoma, Oregon, Rhode Island, South Dakota, Texas, Utah, and Virginia. Washington DC also has a law in place. Two additional states, New York and California, have passed legislation in the House and Senate and the bills are on the governor's desk. Additional legislation is now considered and moving forward in other states including Hawaii, Maine, Michigan, Ohio, and Pennsylvania.

EPILOGUE

Zackery Lystedt rose from his wheelchair and took a few steps with a cane on the stage with his schoolmates at their high school commencement in June 2011. Although still formally enrolled in high school, he is planning to attend a couple of classes at a local community college this year, under his Individual Education Plan. Zack continues to work diligently on his rehabilitation therapy every day as well, hoping to improve his hemiplegia, spasticity, and cognitive skills.

He maintains an inspiring sense of humor and still loves to watch football with his parents. Zack enjoys being with his friends and remains active with the use of social media; he was even elected Prom King this year. Zack has started his first job at Seattle Seahawks training camp, and, in his words, is now a working man. Zackery's parents continue to support his recovery efforts and they remain committed to advocating for sports safety through proper concussion management.

REFERENCES

1. Gilchrist J, Thomas KE, Wald M, et al. Non fatal traumatic brain injuries from sports and recreation activities-the United States, 2001–2005. MMWR Morb Mortal Wkly Rep 2007;56(29):733-7.
2. Wiersma LD, Sherman CP. Volunteer youth sports coach's perspectives of coaching education/certification and parental codes of conduct. Res Q Exerc Sport 2005;76(3):324-38.

Index

Note: Page numbers of article titles are in **boldface** type.

A

Activation
  impaired/abnormal
    after TBI, 580–582
Alzheimer disease
  concussion and, 690
β-Amyloid deposits
  concussion in youth and, 588–589
Athletic participation
  after concussion, 692–693
Axonal injury
  concussion in youth and, 585–587

B

Balance disturbances
  after concussion in youth, 675–676
Balance Error Scoring System (BESS)
  stances for
    in concussion assessment, 611–614
Baseball
  youth concussion in, 567–568
Basketball
  youth concussion in, 568–569
Behavior
  concussion effects on, 688–689
BESS. *See* Balance Error Scoring System (BESS)

C

CBF. *See* Cerebral blood flow (CBF)
Cerebral blood flow (CBF)
  alterations in
    concussion in youth and, 578
Cerebrospinal fluid (CSF) markers
  of repetitive head trauma, 589
Cheerleading
  youth concussion in, 569
Chronic traumatic encephalopathy (CTE)
  after concussion, 626, 690–691
    in youth, 587–590
      β-amyloid deposits in, 588–589
      CSF markers of repetitive head trauma, 589

Phys Med Rehabil Clin N Am 22 (2011) 729–737
doi:10.1016/S1047-9651(11)00091-X
1047-9651/11/$ – see front matter © 2011 Elsevier Inc. All rights reserved.

United States Postal Service

Statement of Ownership, Management, and Circulation
(All Periodicals Publications Except Requestor Publications)

1. Publication Title
Physical Medicine and Rehabilitation Clinics of North America

2. Publication Number 0 0 9 - 2 4 3

3. Filing Date 9/16/11

4. Issue Frequency Feb, May, Aug, Nov

5. Number of Issues Published Annually 4

6. Annual Subscription Price $230.00

7. Complete Mailing Address of Known Office of Publication (Not printer) (Street, city, county, state, and ZIP+4®)
Elsevier Inc.
360 Park Avenue South
New York, NY 10010-1710

Contact Person Stephen Bushing

Telephone (Include area code) 215-239-3688

8. Complete Mailing Address of Headquarters or General Business Office of Publisher (Not printer)
Elsevier Inc., 360 Park Avenue South, New York, NY 10010-1710

9. Full Names and Complete Mailing Addresses of Publisher, Editor, and Managing Editor (Do not leave blank)

Publisher (Name and complete mailing address)
Kim Murphy, Elsevier, Inc., 1600 John F. Kennedy Blvd. Suite 1800, Philadelphia, PA 19103-2899

Editor (Name and complete mailing address)
David Parsons, Elsevier, Inc., 1600 John F. Kennedy Blvd. Suite 1800, Philadelphia, PA 19103-2899

Managing Editor (Name and complete mailing address)
Barbara Cohen-Kligerman, Elsevier, Inc., 1600 John F. Kennedy Blvd. Suite 1800, Philadelphia, PA 19103-2899

10. Owner (Do not leave blank. If the publication is owned by a corporation, give the name and address of the corporation immediately followed by the names and addresses of all stockholders owning or holding 1 percent or more of the total amount of stock. If not owned by a corporation, give the names and addresses of the individual owners. If owned by a partnership or other unincorporated firm, give its name and address as well as those of each individual owner. If the publication is published by a nonprofit organization, give its name and address.)

Full Name	Complete Mailing Address
Wholly owned subsidiary of	4520 East-West Highway
Reed/Elsevier, US holdings	Bethesda, MD 20814

11. Known Bondholders, Mortgagees, and Other Security Holders Owning or Holding 1 Percent or More of Total Amount of Bonds, Mortgages, or Other Securities. If none, check box ☐ None

Full Name	Complete Mailing Address
N/A	

12. Tax Status (For completion by nonprofit organizations authorized to mail at nonprofit rates) (Check one)
The purpose, function, and nonprofit status of this organization and the exempt status for federal income tax purposes:
☐ Has Not Changed During Preceding 12 Months
☐ Has Changed During Preceding 12 Months (Publisher must submit explanation of change with this statement)

PS Form 3526, September 2007 (Page 1 of 3 (Instructions Page 3)) PSN 7530-01-000-9931 PRIVACY NOTICE: See our Privacy policy in www.usps.com

---

13. Publication Title
Physical Medicine and Rehabilitation Clinics of North America

14. Issue Date for Circulation Data Below
August 2011

15. Extent and Nature of Circulation

		Average No. Copies Each Issue During Preceding 12 Months	No. Copies of Single Issue Published Nearest to Filing Date
a. Total Number of Copies (Net press run)		1220	1000
b. Paid Circulation (By Mail and Outside the Mail)	(1) Mailed Outside-County Paid Subscriptions Stated on PS Form 3541. (Include paid distribution above nominal rate, advertiser's proof copies, and exchange copies)	562	541
	(2) Mailed In-County Paid Subscriptions Stated on PS Form 3541 (Include paid distribution above nominal rate, advertiser's proof copies, and exchange copies)		
	(3) Paid Distribution Outside the Mails Including Sales Through Dealers and Carriers, Street Vendors, Counter Sales, and Other Paid Distribution Outside USPS®	169	193
	(4) Paid Distribution by Other Classes Mailed Through the USPS (e.g. First-Class Mail®)		
c. Total Paid Distribution (Sum of 15b (1), (2), (3), and (4))	▲	731	734
d. Free or Nominal Rate Distribution (By Mail and Outside the Mail)	(1) Free or Nominal Rate Outside-County Copies Included on PS Form 3541	64	60
	(2) Free or Nominal Rate In-County Copies Included on PS Form 3541		
	(3) Free or Nominal Rate Copies Mailed at Other Classes Through the USPS (e.g. First-Class Mail)		
	(4) Free or Nominal Rate Distribution Outside the Mail (Carriers or other means)		
e. Total Free or Nominal Rate Distribution (Sum of 15d (1), (2), (3) and (4))	▲	64	60
f. Total Distribution (Sum of 15c and 15e)	▲	795	794
g. Copies not Distributed (See instructions to publishers #4 (page #3))	▲	425	206
h. Total (Sum of 15f and g)	▲	1220	1000
i. Percent Paid (15c divided by 15f times 100)		91.95%	92.44%

16. Publication of Statement of Ownership
☐ If the publication is a general publication, publication of this statement is required. Will be printed in the November 2011 issue of this publication. ☐ Publication not required

17. Signature and Title of Editor, Publisher, Business Manager, or Owner

Stephen R. Bushing
Stephen R. Bushing - Inventory Distribution Coordinator

Date September 16, 2011

I certify that all information furnished on this form is true and complete. I understand that anyone who furnishes false or misleading information on this form or who omits material or information requested on the form may be subject to criminal sanctions (including fines and imprisonment) and/or civil sanctions (including civil penalties).

PS Form 3526, September 2007 (Page 2 of 3)

Moving?

Make sure your subscription moves with you!

To notify us of your new address, find your **Clinics Account Number** (located on your mailing label above your name), and contact customer service at:

Email: journalscustomerservice-usa@elsevier.com

800-654-2452 (subscribers in the U.S. & Canada)
314-447-8871 (subscribers outside of the U.S. & Canada)

Fax number: 314-447-8029

Elsevier Health Sciences Division
Subscription Customer Service
3251 Riverport Lane
Maryland Heights, MO 63043

*To ensure uninterrupted delivery of your subscription, please notify us at least 4 weeks in advance of move.

Printed and bound by CPI Group (UK) Ltd, Croydon, CR0 4YY

03/10/2024

01040439-0018